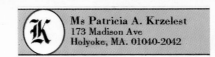

Ms Patricia A. Krzelest
173 Madison Ave
Holyoke, MA. 01040-2042

S0-BDN-068

The process of STAFF DEVELOPMENT

components for change

The process of
STAFF DEVELOPMENT

components for change

HELEN M. TOBIN, R.N., M.S.N.

Director, Centralized Staff Development, University
Hospitals of Cleveland; Associate Clinical Professor,
Frances Payne Bolton School of Nursing,
Case Western Reserve University, Cleveland, Ohio

PAT S. YODER, R.N., M.S.N.

Formerly Assistant Director of Nursing, Mount Clemens
General Hospital, Mount Clemens, Michigan

PEGGY K. HULL, R.N., M.A.

Director, Staff Development, Ohio State University
Hospitals; Instructor, Ohio State University School
of Nursing, Columbus, Ohio

BARBARA CLARK SCOTT, R.N., M.A.

Director of Nursing,
Boca Raton Community Hospital,
Boca Raton, Florida

with 21 illustrations

The C. V. Mosby Company

SAINT LOUIS   1974

Copyright © 1974 by The C. V. Mosby Company

All rights reserved. No part of this book may be
reproduced in any manner without written permission
of the publisher.

Printed in the United States of America

Distributed in Great Britain by Henry Kimpton, London

Library of Congress Cataloging in Publication Data
Main entry under title:

The process of staff development.

   1. Nurses and nursing—Study and teaching.
I. Tobin, Helen M., 1922-
RT71.P86   658.31′24   73-13998
ISBN 0-8016-4995-1

W/S/B 9 8 7 6 5 4 3 2 1

CONTRIBUTORS

Drusilla Poole, R.N., Ph.D. (Colonel, ANC)

Associate Professor,
University of Maryland School of Nursing;
Director, Walter Reed Army Institute of Nursing,
Washington, D. C.

Dorothy H. Coye, R.N., M.S.N.

Director of Nursing Education,
William Beaumont Hospital,
Royal Oak, Michigan

**To our families and friends
and staff development educators**

PREFACE

This book could be called "Getting It All Together," because that is our intent. In December, 1968, the need for some guidelines for staff development was identified. As we started writing guidelines, we found some information was not in print and some was obscure. Thus what started to be a small task developed into a major effort.

As the whole continuing education effort is being discussed and examined by various groups within the profession at the state and national level, it becomes increasingly important to define parameters of the issue and to determine the purpose of continuing education.

One segment of the continuing education effort occurs within the agency. Formerly referred to as in-service education, staff development is realizing new significance as the numbers and types of health care workers undergo major changes. Additionally, there now are explicit statements that define certain agencies' responsibilities for providing appropriate educational offerings as well as those that define the responsibilities of practitioners for participating in educational offerings.

The process of staff development involves three major aspects: input, process, and output. Various factors relating to these three areas appear throughout this book. The process is identified in relation to nursing within health care agencies, but the concepts are applicable to other groups.

The subtitle, *Components for Change*, indicates the significance of the process, because changing behavior is the focus of staff development. If there were no discrepancies between what is demonstrated and what is desired, it would be questionable if staff development education were needed. Realistically, we know that many discrepancies do exist and that some are priority matters for improving the care nursing's clients receive. The components involved in the process lead toward the ultimate goal of improved health care to consumers.

The intent of this book is not to provide a text of one viewpoint, but rather to examine the development, process, and concepts of staff development education and its relationship to the overall continuing education effort. We have included a history of staff development and the perspective of today's continuing education efforts as well as concepts about motivation and adult learning, two of the essential considerations in pursuing staff development. Additionally, we have attempted to include various considerations to be evaluated in different situations. Each aspect in this book offers guidelines for use in establishing or altering staff development education within an agency. Depending on available resources, implementation can be modified to meet specific needs within various agencies.

This book is intended primarily for staff development educators as a guide to developing or revising their efforts within the agency. It is useful, also, to administrators of nursing services in planning for staff development. Additionally, it may prove interesting to educators in schools of nursing in meeting their own staff development needs as well as in understanding the process to which their graduates should be exposed. How it is used depends primarily on the philosophy of each agency and the nursing department and organization of the staff development effort. It is important for each user of this book to apply the information within the context of the employing agency.

Many concepts are expressed in this book. If the readers can meet most of the key objectives provided in the text, they will have a base for implementing the concepts expressed here. Modifying approaches yields different outcomes, but the outcomes should be a desirable change in behavior.

Without the understanding and help of our families and friends, we would have been unable to complete this publication. We thank our colleagues for the stimulating discussions that have assisted in the development of this book. We appreciate the extreme helpfulness of Geraldine Mink, Assistant Professor of Nursing (Library Methodology), Frances Payne Bolton School of Nursing, Case Western Reserve University, and Head of References, Cleveland Health Sciences Library, for reading the manuscript. Finally, we appreciate the contributions of Drusilla Poole and Dorothy H. Coye.

Helen M. Tobin
Pat S. Yoder
Peggy K. Hull
Barbara Clark Scott

CONTENTS

1

Continuing education and staff development

Let us never consider ourselves finished nurses.

FLORENCE NIGHTINGALE

Since the beginning of time, there has always been something new to learn. How we learn and how others know that we learn have become increasingly important. As the demand for public accountability has increased, evaluating performance on the job has become more important to employers. Higher costs of health care, for example, have encouraged administrators to look closely at individual performances to justify maintaining persons in their present positions, advancing them to other positions, or terminating their employment. An understanding of the concepts of andragogy (adult learning) has changed the way in which agencies have offered learning opportunities. No longer do we view a once-a-month lecture as sufficient.

Historically, in-service education has long been a part of hospital nursing services. It has served to identify and meet learning needs. Although some hospitals still focus all their energies on orientation-skill training services, many have developed additional offerings to meet their employees' needs. Today there are hospitals that, through the sharing of both personnel and equipment, are better utilizing their resources.

Having taken a strong interest in community education, nursing sought to identify the learning needs of those within its ranks who had not had prior exposure to community health nursing. As a result, nursing was better able to give families, new mothers, the sick, and the well a more comprehensive understanding of health and illness. Yet we hear from others that staff development is "new."

Social forces, the differences between the three types of basic nursing education programs, and the motivation to be employed within a particular agency have contributed to the change in what agencies offer in learning experiences.[1] For many people, financial security is not the only goal to be achieved; rather, rewards are also sought in the areas of professional and personal development.

The concept of staff development may not be as new as the term. Originally, continuing education was carried out within the confines of the institution. However, the ever-increasing rate of technological discovery has drastically altered the situation; it is now estimated that the half-life of science and technology affecting nursing care methods is between three to five years. Because of the vast amount of knowledge to be learned, it has become necessary that various educational institutions, professional and voluntary organizations, and health care agencies be more actively involved in providing continued learning opportunities.[2,3] Thus the concept of "in-service education" (within the agency) has been transformed into that of "staff development" (within and outside the agency).

Patient education has also taken on new dimensions. Formalized classes are being offered to deal with the increased complexity of health problems, with the goal of involving clients in their care so that realistic, workable plans may be developed.

In addition, we must also take into account the large numbers of health workers now involved in health care agencies. At least 200

1

separate careers have been identified for persons interested in the health care field. All of these health workers have learning needs peculiar to their own work as well as the need for a general understanding of the other areas of the health care system. Indeed, even the traditional role of the physician has undergone such change that some people do not now understand what the parameters of that profession are.

CONTINUING EDUCATION

The overall problem of continuing education has been explored by various groups. The American Nurses' Association in 1967 identified three distinct areas of education—formal academic study, continuing education, and independent learning.[4] Although there are preparatory programs of differing quality and type, one common factor is that none ensure that practitioners will maintain competency throughout their careers. Also in 1967 the National Advisory Commission on Health Manpower called for examining relicensure practices and continuing education.[5] The Department of Health, Education, and Welfare in its *Report on Licensure and Related Health Personnel Credentialing* discussed the aspect of continuing education in relation to combating professional obsolescence.[6] Although the need for continuing education is great, there are logistical problems that must be dealt with if mandatory continuing education is to be considered.

The National Commission for the Study of Nursing and Nursing Education has suggested that the problems of continuing education in nursing may be greater than in other professions because of the variety of preservice educational programs used in the preparation of registered nurses.[7] The full report, *An Abstract for Action,* calls for various steps to be taken to provide continuing education for the hundreds of thousands of registered nurses in this country.[8] Qualified leaders and organizational support are regarded as being of primary importance for the achievement of this end.

Is there a need for concerted efforts to provide continuing education and to encourage individuals to participate? According to a report from the Western Interstate Commission for Higher Education, the answer is an obvious one. From WICHE's projections the assumption is made that "... more than 70 percent of practicing nurses may not be pursuing planned programs to increase their competence as practitioners."[9] Additionally, the need has been recognized organizationally since 1969 when a group of nurses involved in continuing education, primarily university based, met at the National Conference on Continuing Education for Nursing. The following meetings have focused on the various issues involving nursing and continuing education. Evidence of concern with continuing education appears more frequently in recent nursing literature, especially the *Journal of Continuing Education in Nursing.* The need has been well documented.

In order to meet the learning needs of nurses, we must use all potential resources, one of which is staff development. Thus it is important that we understand what continuing education is and how staff development relates to it.

Continuing education consists of systematic learning experiences designed to build upon preservice knowledge and skills. It includes an organized, planned program and an independent endeavor on the part of the learner. It is distinguished from academic pursuits in that no formal credit is granted and the acquisition of a higher degree is not the goal. Simply stated it refers to structured, nonacademic learning after completion of a basic program, whereas continued learning includes academic advancement as well as those endeavors identified as continuing education and casual learning. Some learning is not systematic and therefore would not be defined as continuing education; for example, while two nurses may expand each other's knowledge by presenting divergent viewpoints, it is not a result of a planned or systematic activity. However, attending a related seminar would represent continuing education as well as continued learning. Additionally, they may seek readings or other self-instructional methods to continue learning in a systematic manner.

If we view continuing education as a whole, for example, a circle with a variety of learning segments, we can begin to see how staff development relates to the total picture. Fig. 1-1 shows staff development as a part of the total learning effort, that part which is oriented toward improvement of performance at work.° In order to maximize learning, staff development draws on other areas that are viewed as relevant to the performance at work. Traditionally, the agency attempted to meet needs through in-agency offerings. Thus in-service was viewed as the whole effort. The term "staff development," however, encompasses instruction outside the agency designed to supplement in-service learning, thus providing a broader base of educational opportunities to enhance learning. If a registered nurse

°Orientation within staff development is not viewed as an integral part of continuing education, but rather as a basic requirement for functioning in a given position.

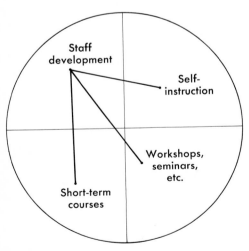

Fig. 1-1. Staff development within continuing education. The total continuing education effort includes a variety of ways to improve knowledge. The staff development segment not only contributes a basic portion but also draws on other areas to improve the performance of employees.

who is an adult cardiac care specialist enrolls in a short-term "infant care" course, it may be considered continuing education, but it is not staff development because the course would not contribute directly to performance at work.

When agencies use the staff development approach, someone must review the "outside" activities and evaluate the contributions a particular offering will make to the agency. In the preceding example the agency would receive little benefit in the way of improved nursing care because this nurse does not work with infants. It would be far better to send a nurse who worked with infants to this course if specific, dynamic returns are expected.

STAFF DEVELOPMENT

Staff development includes both formal and informal learning activities that relate to the employee's role and that take place either within or outside the agency. This means that any effort to improve an employee's skills and knowledge should be considered continued learning.

Staff development differs from in-service education, as evidenced in the following definition: in-service education is that part of continued learning which the agency offers to increase the employees' skills and knowledge in relation to the role expectations. As the word "in-service" implies, this learning occurs *within* the service agency.

The broader concept of staff development encompasses two major components—orientation and continuing education. Briefly, orientation is the attempt to make new employees aware of policies, procedures, philosophies, purposes, personnel benefits, and position requirements. It may include such facets as skill training, for example, nurse assistants training courses and defibrillation drills. It also may include instruction in leadership skills, for instance, providing potential candidates for a head nurse position with basic knowledge for fulfilling the role expectations.

Continuing education *within staff development* should provide personnel with the opportunity to learn new knowledge and skills, review and add to knowledge already gained, investigate new approaches in nursing, and strengthen their clinical competencies. For example, the fostering of innovative and creative approaches to nursing care of patients might be undertaken for the purpose of achieving more effective behavior in nursing practice, which improves the quality of patient care and leads to increased job satisfaction. Continuing education encompasses all efforts (other than orientation) to maintain and improve the abilities of employees. Thus skill training and leadership development are a part of continuing education also, because they provide additional knowledge and skills for those persons who have had no previous exposure to this content.

Process of staff development

Either component of staff development is approached in the same manner. The process used to plan, conduct, and evaluate staff development should allow for adherence to standards as well as recognition of individual needs. Fig. 1-2 represents the process of staff development. Even though a sequential approach is used, each factor is interrelated with all others to the extent that the process is dynamic. Alteration of one factor usually affects the others.

The three phases—input, process, and output—are essential to the overall goal of changed behavior. *Input* factors represent the "givens" in the process and are divided into two main segments, organizational and individual. Within the organizational factors there are some rather delimiting items. Standards of care, whether developed by the agency or by the profession, are a basis for the formulation of overall goals. Both the organizational and individual factors define certain parameters for the agency and give direction to the staff development process. Role expectations for various employees are identified to determine how everyone should work together to achieve the agency's goals. These expectations describe the required behaviors of individuals

in a given position, thus setting criteria by which individuals are judged. Without role expectations it is difficult, if not impossible, to judge the output and to have an effective process. Finally, the resources available should be considered in order to obtain realistic objectives and learning experiences. While the goals of the agency may require certain performance behaviors, there may not be adequate resources available with which to achieve these goals. Thus additional resources need to be considered.

The individual factors pertain to the learners and determine the material to be offered. Learner profiles identify characteristics, learning styles, goals, and needs. Probably the most significant factor for the learners is that concerning "goals." What the new or current employees want to gain from their experiences within the agency greatly influences what and how they will learn. If their goals coincide with the agency's expectations, there is concurrence of needs. If not, there is a dichotomy. "Needs," then, are most important to the development of the process, and they imply specific modifications for the learning offering. (In the planning stage for orientation it may be necessary to make some generalizations about the anticipated group until the individuals have the opportunity to identify their goals and needs.) The learning offering should represent what is needed in terms of knowledge, skills, and attitudes. There is core learning, which is basic to a given group in terms of expected behaviors, and there is career learning, which expands the "basics" into long-range offerings. All these factors are so interrelated that the process may not be effective if one aspect is neglected.

Within the context of the climate and planning mechanism, the next step, *process*, begins. Climate setting appears in two phases of the process—planning and implementation. In planning one must consider the climate within the agency in order to identify needs and to design a plan to meet these needs. In implementation, climate setting is once again emphasized in order to establish the most con-

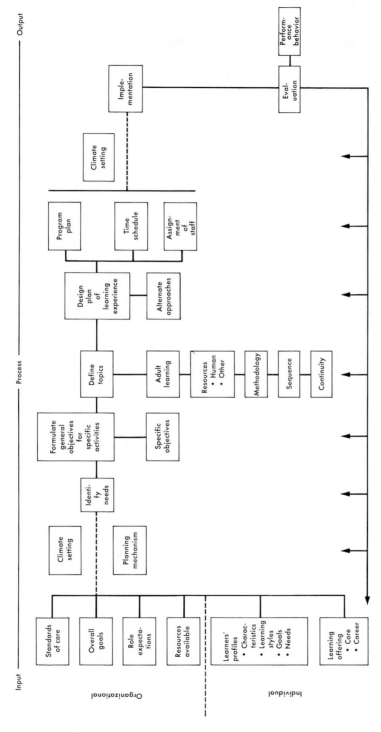

Fig. 1-2. Staff development process. The staff development process is a step-by-step approach that is interrelated and ongoing. Evaluation is incorporated throughout the process.

ducive atmosphere for learning. Although climate setting is not a specific step, as denoted in Fig. 1-2 by the broken line, it influences the rest of the process.

The planning mechanism represents the organization and administration of the staff development effort (Chapter 5). The rest of the process is developed within the framework of a centralized and/or decentralized approach.

Identification of needs is based on the input and influenced by the climate and planning mechanism. For example, concurrence of agency and individual goals usually results in fewer needs than when a dichotomy exists. Each of the input factors influences what is identified as a "need." These may be identified by the staff development educator, by clinical nursing personnel, or by a committee, depending on the mechanism within the agency. Chapter 7 describes ways in which needs can be identified.

After particular needs are identified, they are translated into general and specific objectives, as described in Chapter 6. These objectives establish an evaluation mechanism and guide the development of a learning experience. If the objectives are well defined and behaviorally oriented, it is likely that evaluation will be easier. The specific topics are based on these objectives. We must consider concepts of adult learning in defining topics (Chapter 3) as well as in determining the individual input factors. Each of the factors (adult learning, resources, methodology, sequence, and continuity) influences how the topic is defined. For example, the sequence of topics might allow for core content for various employees and branched content for specific groups.

The plan of learning experiences describes how the objectives are going to be met (Chapter 8). In designing the plan, various approaches are considered: one is selected and the others are retained as alternatives. In designing the program, three aspects must be defined in order to allow for realistic implementation. Most significantly, the program plan is developed. This should describe the specific content and activities involved in the learning offering. Next, time and staff assignment are considered. In order to develop the time schedule, several factors need to be considered (Chapter 9). Such factors as availability of the learners and the assigning of staff are crucial to the successful implementation of the program. Although there are a variety of ways to assign the staff, the best method is to consider who is most qualified for each position. Individuals could be assigned by shifts, type of personnel, components, or clinical expertise.

Again, climate setting is significant in the implementation phase. For example, how the learners are greeted may influence how receptive they will be to a given program. Implementation ultimately results in evaluation and output. As identified in Fig. 1-2, evaluation is a continuous process and is important at each and every step, being particularly crucial to future planning (Chapter 10).

The third phase, *output,* is demonstrated in performance behaviors, which should identify the success or failure of the staff development effort. As stated earlier, the purpose of staff development is change in behavior; thus, if no change is seen or the change is not desirable, the output is not what was expected and there was an error made in determining input or in using the process. The success of the process relates directly to the effort used in assessing, developing, and effecting each step.

IMPACT OF CONTINUING EDUCATION

Having established a frame of reference, we may now examine statements of the profession and the standards of regulatory or accrediting bodies that are supportive of continued learning.

In 1965 the American Nurses' Association stated, "The nursing department provides training programs and opportunities for staff development."[10] Six assessment factors are identified for use as measures of attainment.

  a. Training programs are provided for auxiliary nursing personnel to enable them

to acquire needed knowledge and skills and to help them adjust to their new environment.
b. Programs for staff development utilize educational resources inside and outside the health care facility.
c. Selected staff members are encouraged to prepare themselves for greater responsibility in nursing.
d. Plans are developed in advance to prepare selected personnel to function in new or expanded nursing care programs.
e. Staff members are encouraged to develop avocational interests and aptitudes.
f. The health care facility provides a library of books and current periodicals which nursing service personnel are encouraged to use.°

Where continued learning efforts have real impact, however, is in law or accreditation standards. For example, in 1970 the Joint Commission for Accreditation of Hospitals proposed, "There shall be continuing training programs and educational opportunities for the development of nursing personnel."[11] The statement goes on to cite a variety of factors that should be assessed during the accreditation process.

Although some states have recognized efforts in continuing education, primarily through state nurses' associations, it was not until 1971 that California became the first state to make proof of continuing education for registered nurses and licensed practical nurses a requirement for relicensure. This law established a council to develop standards in such a way as to provide alternatives to licensees. "Such alternatives include, but are not limited to, academic studies, inservice education, institutes, seminars, lectures, conferences, workshops, extension studies, and home-study programs."[12] Suddenly, the "nice, extra effort" became a matter of necessity: we must provide continuing learning experiences and keep an accurate record of them.

As recently as 1973, the American Nurses'

°American Nurses' Association: Standards for organized nursing services, Kansas City, Mo., 1965. The Association. Reprinted with permission.

Association revised its statement[13] regarding staff development as follows:

The nursing administration provides programs for orientation and continued learning of nursing personnel.

Guidelines

a. Orientation programs are offered to all newly employed personnel with content including but not limited to:
 1. Philosophy and objectives of the health care organization and nursing service
 2. Personnel policies
 3. Job descriptions
 4. Work environment
 5. Clinical practice policies and procedures
 6. Operational policies and procedures
b. Nursing administration shares responsibility with individual practitioners and other health care agencies to promote continuous learning experiences which insure current knowledge and practice.
c. A program for performance evaluation of all nursing staff is operational.°

As evidenced by the preceding standards, statements, and reports, continuing education is here to stay. Within continuing education, staff development has become more crucial to health care agencies as they attempt to meet the constant needs of their employees to maintain and improve their knowledge and skills, so that they may provide better care for the consumers. In the past, continuing education and staff development have been recognized as desirable assets, but only in recent years have real strides been made to provide both to a wider population of health workers. The groundwork laid in the past prepares us for the future.

°American Nurses' Association: Standards for nursing services, Kansas City, Mo., 1973, The Association. Reprinted with permission.

REFERENCES
1. Tobin, H. M., and Wengerd, J. S.: What makes a staff development program work? Am. J. Nurs. **71:** 940, 1971.
2. Yoder, P. S.: Planning for learning through the pro-

fessional association, J. Cont. Educ. Nurs. **3**(5):22, 1972.

3. Clark, B. J.: Formulating an assembly of staff development educators, J. Cont. Educ. Nurs. **3**(5):27, 1972.
4. American Nurses' Association: Avenues for continued learning, Kansas City, Mo., 1967, The Association.
5. Report of the National Advisory Commission on Health Manpower, Washington, D. C., 1967, U. S. Government Printing Office.
6. Department of Health, Education, and Welfare: Report on licensure and related health personnel credentialing, Washington, D. C., 1971, U. S. Government Printing Office.
7. Lysaught, J. P.: Continuing education: necessity and opportunity, J. Cont. Educ. Nurs. **1**(3):5, 1970.
8. An abstract for action; report of the National Commission for the Study of Nursing and Nursing Education, New York, 1970, McGraw-Hill Book Co.
9. Western Interstate Commission for Higher Education: Continuing education in nursing, Boulder, Colo., 1969, The Commission.
10. American Nurses' Association: Standards for organized nursing services, Kansas City, Mo., 1965, The Association.
11. Joint Commission for Accreditation of Hospitals: Accreditation manual, Chicago, 1970, The Commission.
12. California State Assembly Bill No. 449, Chapter 1516.
13. American Nurses' Association: Standards for nursing services, Kansas City, Mo., 1973, The Association.

BIBLIOGRAPHY

Allison, E. W.: Mandatory continuing education? Am. J. Nurs. **73**:413, 1973.

American Nurses' Association: Statement of beliefs on inservice education and functions and qualifications for inservice educators, New York, 1966, The Association.

Brown, C. R., and Uhl, H. S. M.: Mandatory continuing education: sense or nonsense? J.A.M.A., **213**:1660, 1970.

Cooper, S. S.: Mandatory continuing education, Am. J. Nurs. **73**:442, 1973.

Coye, D. H.: What is continuing education in nursing service? Supervisor Nurse **1**(6):36, 1970.

Gibbs, G. E.: Will continuing education be required for license renewal? Am. J. Nurs. **71**:2175, 1971.

Hayter, J.: Individual responsibility for continuing education, J. Cont. Educ. Nurs. **3**(6):31, 1972.

Hornback, M. S.: Continuing education—whose responsibility? J. Cont. Educ. Nurs. **2**(4):9, 1971.

Houle, C. O.: The comparative study of continuing professional education, J. Cont. Educ. Nurs. **3**(3):4, 1972.

Huber, C.: Continuing education: voluntary or mandatory? In Three challenges to the nursing profession, Kansas City, Mo., 1972, American Nurses' Association.

McGriff, E. P.: A case for mandatory continuing education in nursing, Nurs. Outlook **20**:712, 1972.

National Conference on Continuing Education in Nursing: Critical issues in continuing education in nursing, Madison, 1972, University of Wisconsin Press.

Nattress, L. W.: Continuing education for the professions in the United States, Convergence **3**(4):42, 1970.

Nylan, M. S., et al.: An interprofessional approach to continuing education in the health sciences, J. Cont. Educ. Nurs. **2**(4):21, 1971.

Ohliger, J.: Accent on social philosophy: lifelong learning—voluntary or compulsory? Adult leadership **17**(3):124, 1968.

Pluckhan, M. L., Peltier, Sr. R., and Spicher, E.: Meeting the challenge: coordination and facilitation of statewide continuing education for nurses through interdisciplinary and interagency action, J. Cont. Educ. Nurs. **4**(1):22, 1973.

Spector, A. F.: The American Nurses' Association and continuing education, J. Cont. Educ. Nurs. **2**(2):41, 1971.

2 History of staff development

DRUSILLA POOLE

The best prophet of the future is the past.
JOHN SHERMAN

The historical sequence of the development of the basic components for staff development programs in nursing cannot be divorced from the events that were taking place in the world around it. The expansion of these components has been an ongoing process throughout this century, paralleling the advances made in nursing as a whole. It is possible to explain the growth in the scope of staff development by historical review. Such a review will provide a basis for a better understanding of the current definition of staff development and the trends within this type of educational experience for nursing service personnel.

In 1928 Pfefferkorn,[1] in an historical review of in-service education, wrote that although in-service education had long been present in nursing, it was still in its infancy. Since that time there have been few articles on the subject. In an unpublished paper presented in San Francisco in 1957 on the history of in-service education, Lulu Wolf Hassenplug described, in part, the same historical sequence that will be referred to in this discussion.

R. Louise McManus[2] once stated that the amount and kind of emphasis now being placed on in-service education could not and would not have occurred in any century prior to the twentieth. The importance of the worker and his rights are ideas unique to this century. A contemporary administrator's concerns include the quality of service rendered by a worker as well as what happens to the worker while giving the service. Miller[3] said that the recognition of human resources as our most valuable asset is the primary cause of the current emphasis on the worker. Perhaps the greatest force in bringing about special approaches to the training of large numbers of unskilled workers were the demands made by the two world wars on American industry. The success or failure of the various management techniques that were implemented to ensure the maximum contribution of these workers to industry provides a source of valuable data to be used in the study and analysis of staff development techniques. Following World War II, management became a speciality and the position of training director was created within this field. Although direct translation of industrial practices is not deemed feasible, much can be gained by highly selective borrowing and skillful application of proved programs to the problems of nursing services.

Many who work in staff development regard adult education as a more widespread and adaptable frame of reference. This century has fostered the concept of a "second chance for all." On a phenomenal scale adults are resuming their educations in all kinds of programs under the auspices of different organizations. Even more significant has been the impact of the concept of adult education as

9

"lifetime learning."[4] The rapidity of change, scientific advances, and growth in technology have forced us to recognize that a limited period of education is not sufficient in this century. The essentiality of adult learning has lessened the resistance to continuing education and has provided the perfect setting for expanding the scope and purpose of in-service education.

Turning our attention to organized nursing services in the postwar period, we find that changes were taking place. Nursing was responsive and receptive to in-service education as a form of adult education and as a component of management. Gradually, organized nursing services began to realize the need for directors of in-service education. The number of these positions increased slowly. The well-defined duties of the educational directors in the Veterans Administration hospitals were an exception to the usual confusion that existed in most hospitals, where an educational director had combined duties in a school of nursing and in a nursing service. The military educational coordinator was utilized in a variety of ways, depending on the chief nurse's concept of in-service education. The role of the in-service education director is still being clarified.

A milestone was reached when directors of nursing in hospitals and agencies began to set up separate departments for in-service education and to assign responsibility to assistant directors.[5] As an increasing number of hospitals gave status and scope to full-time positions for staff development education, academic preparation for this position became necessary. In response to this need the Kellogg Foundation in 1950 included the following objectives in its program for the improvement of nursing services: to expand the scope of extension courses to nursing service administration, to enlarge curriculum offerings of in-service education for nurses employed in hospitals, to design programs to upgrade nursing practice, and to keep nurses informed of new developments in the field of nursing.[6] These objectives were agreed upon by four-teen universities. Since that time there has been some growth in the number of academic programs offering study in in-service education. Because of this new emphasis there have been improvements in the types of in-service programs, the performance of directors, and the acceptance of staff development objectives as a function of nursing administration.

How did these events and their historical setting affect our current perception of staff development as an integral part of nursing service administration and supervision? When staff development programs are considered essential to the recruitment and retention of new nurses in a particular practice setting, what are the basic components one expects to find in a comprehensive program? What is the definition of staff development? The answers to these questions can be formulated by examining the past.

The depression of the 1920's and 1930's forced large numbers of nurses, for the first time in the history of the profession, to move from individual practices to hospital services.[7] The need to ease this transition for both the nurses and their administrators resulted in the first organized approach to staff development. This early emphasis was on *orientation*. Professional nurses, new to the hospital setting as staff members, needed to become acquainted with equipment, procedures, and regulations. They had to become accustomed to working with other nurses and caring for groups of patients. It is natural that orientation is still the basic and first component of staff development with which nursing personnel become involved.

The second area of emphasis evolved from expressed needs for improvement in nursing practice. After their initial orientation, nurses began to be concerned about their on-the-job skills. The 1930's and 1940's were characterized by great efforts in *skill training*. The most popular programs for improving nursing care were in certain clinical speciality areas and reflected the enormous strides that were being made in technical knowledge and skills. Some of our outstanding nursing specialists of today had their interest in a particular specialty aroused by workshops and short courses. Skill training needs were further stressed by conditions brought about by World War II. Refresher courses were set up for the large number of previously inactive nurses who returned to duty in hospitals. On-the-job training programs of all kinds were started for volunteers during this period. The entrance of the non-professional nursing worker and the beginning of the team concept increased the skill training needs in hospitals.[8] This aspect of in-service education (skill training) is still one of the most popular and interesting of our nursing service programs. However, the concept of in-service training has been expanded to include skills other than the manual and technical ones.

In the 1940's and 1950's nurses became concerned with self-evaluation. They began to examine their own qualifications, both personal and professional, against the standards being set by the profession. There was a tremendous upsurge in educational activities as academic requirements of the professional were being established.[9] The motivation for *continuing education* and the expansion of the intellectual interests of professional nurses have yet to be completed. There has been phenomenal progress, but the job is never finished. Continuing education has been likened to the care a gardener gives his garden after the seeds have been planted and the young seedlings have appeared. The analogy is a valid one and points to the fact that staff development is truly a continuing process.

The progress in continuing education resulted in the profession's taking a very critical look at the kind of leadership available within nursing. It is a sign of growth when a profession, an organization, or an individual becomes concerned with the caliber of its leadership. In the 1950's and 1960's nursing continued to work to develop *leadership and management skills.* Each generation of nurses looks for those who can qualify for leadership roles and who exemplify the progress that the profession has made. Today's leaders are better

prepared for nursing practice than any who have come before them. They will make significant contributions to the more effective utilization of nursing resources by evaluating the leadership role and their own positions. There is no substitute for professional leadership as the driving force behind improvement of nursing services and nursing education. The progress of the profession has a direct relation to the number of leaders who see those whom they have led surpass them in ability and achievement. Newton[10] described this as the "joy of leadership."

The next emphasis in nursing affecting in-service education in the 1960's was the result of momentum in *research*. Participation in research was the natural outcome of a willingness on the part of nurses to be critical of their practice and to seek a sound and scientific explanation for doing, or for not doing, what they had been taught and what they had observed about nursing. Research is inextricably interwoven with in-service education. Heidgerken[11] stated that in-service education is the vehicle by which the results of research are translated into practice. Nurses should eagerly welcome all opportunities to participate in research, to be knowledgeable in research activities, and to take the findings of research and attempt to use them in their particular fields of nursing. Programs that are designed to assist nursing service personnel in accomplishing these research endeavors is indeed the result of an exciting and powerful new aspect of staff development.[7]

In the 1970's new concerns for nursing and consequently a new emphasis on staff development have emerged. In order that the nursing professionals may work toward becoming true colleagues of other professionals, the basic preparation of practitioners is being moved into educational institutions, and attempts to identify the necessary advanced academic and experiential preparation for leaders continue. When nursing practitioners become more broadly educated, an exciting and challenging era in nursing will begin. That the broadly educated nurse will practice nursing in a different and more effective way is a challenging hypothesis for both nursing education and nursing service. Preservice and staff development programs and curricula are more interdependent today then ever before in nursing history. Decisions as to where essential learning must take place cannot be delayed, and the concept of nursing education as a lifelong continuum is close to becoming a reality.

Perhaps there is no one simple term that can be applied to the nursing concerns of the 1970's. A more clear-cut direction will no doubt evolve, but at the present time there appear to be two points of particular interest— the *personalized professional practice of the nurse* and the *problem of the relevance of the profession.* Its members want nursing to be in the mainstream of society. The old isolationism is intolerable to those who believe that nursing action can make a difference in the health of all people. Nursing is needed beyond the limiting walls of institutions and agencies; nurses must be everywhere. They see people as the aim and center of their work and their caring. There seems to be a vocal rejection of those aspects, however necessary according to established systems, that dilute the directness of care. Nurses want the profession to be relevant to the current scene and the practice to be significant in solving the ills of the world—yes, even beyond that aim, toward the realization of a world that is healthy. They are less awed by technology and more suspicious of its so-called advantages. They trust their own judgment and put great stock in personal competence. They are constructively worried about their world and fearful for its survival. They want skills and knowledge that permit them to move toward goals *they* care about. Old accepted motives, values, systems, and practices are all under attack. Commitments may still be strong, but they are selectively made. The integrity of one's own identity, goals, and talents is sacred. The truly professional member of society is viewed as potentially more self-directing than nurses have traditionally been. Many see this

as one of the very real issues facing today's nurses. They believe that this attitude will differentiate the new generation of nurses from the old. The preparation for and the accommodation of self-directiveness within the currently structured nursing organization necessitate new goals that must effect change at all levels of education. A totally new era in staff development is being born and programs as yet unconceived must become part of nursing in the next decades.

We have traced the story of staff development in nursing through more than half a century. In each decade nursing has demonstrated a responsiveness to the trends and issues characteristic of that decade. And while each period has been different, in sequence each may be seen as part of a pattern. The logical concerns about the growth of the profession may be similar to those of an individual who experiences professional growth: the ever-widening objectives of one's learning move from a relatively self-centered preoccupation with orientation needs and skill deficits to that of continuing education which enables one to assume a questioning attitude toward leadership and to study practice, and then on toward a conceptualization about the professional's role and society's health. The synchronization of educationally sound and stimulating programs with the expanding learning needs of individuals, of groups within a segment of nursing, and of the profession is the real key to the motivation and valuation of staff development and the lesson of its history.

REFERENCES

1. Pfefferkorn, B.: Improvement of the nurse in service—an historical review, Am. J. Nurs.**28:**700, 1928.
2. McManus, R. L.: Unpublished paper presented at In-Service Education Workshop, Medical Field Service School, Fort Sam Houston, Texas, Nov. 29, 1955.
3. Miller, M. A.: Inservice education for hospital nursing personnel, New York, 1958, National League for Nursing, Inc.
4. Pears, R.: The meaning of adult education, Adult Leadership **2:**2, 32, April, 1954.
5. Poole, D.: In-service education reaches a milestone, Am. J. Nurs. **53:**1456, 1953.

6. Miller, M. A.: Trends of in-service education. In Cowan, C., editor: The yearbook of modern nursing, New York, 1956, G. P. Putnam's Sons.

7. Lambertsen, E. C.: Education for nursing leadership, Philadelphia, 1958, J. B. Lippincott Co.

8. Bridgman, M.: Collegiate education for nursing, New York, 1953, Russell Sage Foundation.

9. McManus, R. L.: What colleges and universities offer the practicing nurse, Am. J. Nurs. **54:**1478, 1954.

10. Newton, M. E.: Developing leadership potential, Nurs. Outlook **5:**400, 1957.

11. Heidgerken, L.: In-service education and research, Nurs. Outlook **7:**474, 1959.

3

Adult learning

*If you don't think there's a difference between
training and education, put the word "sex" in front
of the words and determine if you would let your
nine-year-old child take the course.*

ANONYMOUS

To avoid lengthy and sometimes stalemated discussion of the differences between training and education, this chapter is entitled "Adult Learning." Additionally, this title places the focus where it belongs—on how the adult learns rather than on how he is taught.

Adults have always learned, but not always in a systematic fashion. Only in recent years have we recognized the significance of adult learning. Although many books and articles have focused on the unique factors of adult learning, it is only recently that these concepts have been applied in school classrooms.[1] Thus while some of the ideas in this chapter are no longer unique, they remain extremely significant to adult learners.

The purpose of adult learning is to improve one's competency in life. In this context, the question of learning versus schooling is critical. While it is not necessary for an individual to attend school forever, we find that individuals who stop learning soon become stagnant. In the past, knowledge was not changing so rapidly; hence continuing education was not deemed so critical as it is today. In fact, as cited in the first chapter, our knowledge becomes outdated very rapidly.

In the early 1970's Toffler[2] illustrated that we are, in essence, running to stay behind. We cannot be secure in the efforts we make to update our knowledge, because the object of our quest is in a constant state of change.

Therefore lifelong learning is absolutely essential to continued competency. As Stein[3] points out, continuing education is an individual matter as well as a social phenomenon. It is impossible to survive in today's work world with only that knowledge gained in childhood and early adulthood. Stein bases this statement on an article by Mead,[4] which contends that we do not live in the same world into which we were born, and that we will not die in the world in which we worked. Thus we are assured of having continual learning needs.

One of the first efforts in the United States to provide adult learning situations focused on farmers and was essentially *job oriented*, designed to improve farm productivity. This focus (job oriented), involving a majority of organized adult learning efforts, is not the only one. The adult who enrolls in a basic real estate course may be completely removed from that field, but the learning experience will make the individual more competent in personal life should the family home be sold.

Although adult education encompasses more than those learning opportunities that are job oriented, it is this aspect on which staff development educators must focus. In order for staff development educators to facilitate that portion of adult learning which is job oriented, certain key concepts about andragogy must be applied in the program offerings.

ANDRAGOGY

The term "andragogy," which now appears frequently in the literature, has been traced to Alexander Kapp, a German grammar school teacher. In 1833 he used andragogy as distinguished from pedagogy to refer to the normal, natural process of continuing education for adults. Prior to the 1920's much research had been conducted about how learning occurred, but the learners were children, not adults. Perhaps the most well known of the early studies focusing on adults as learners was conducted by Thorndike.[5] This study revealed that adults learned but at a slower rate and in a different manner than children.

Unfortunately, while we know some significant factors relating to adult learning, we continue to violate many of the "rules." For example, Powell[6] states that the adult mind differs from that of an undergraduate or youth as it relates ideas to experience. Yet how many times have we as adults spent the entire day in a continuing education effort such as a lecture where there was no opportunity for participation? Worse yet we may have had difficult seating arrangements, limited breaks, and no writing space! These physical distractions may inhibit the mind and allow for little opportunity to relate ideas to past experiences.

In order to implement a sound program of staff development, it is necessary to have an understanding of some basic differences between andragogy and pedagogy.

DIFFERENCES BETWEEN ANDRAGOGY (TEACHING OF ADULTS) AND PEDAGOGY (TEACHING OF CHILDREN)

Various authors have used different points of reference in their comparisons of pedagogy and andragogy. The following is a brief summary of the comparisons made by three of the principal authors—Kidd, Miller, and Knowles.

Kidd's differentiation[7]

One of the early, nationally recognized writers on adult learning, Kidd compares learning with the art of medicine, which he believes is primarily concerned with preventing further bodily damage and creating a healing environment. In other words adult educators should be more concerned with facilitating learning, providing a climate for learning, and freeing the learner to learn rather than burdening him with structured content and formats. An adult will learn if he is presented with the chance to do so.

Kidd cites four ways in which adult learning situations differ from those of children. The first we are familiar with no matter what our occupation: adults usually find themselves in situations where there is no totally "correct" answer. For instance, the solution of a business problem requires a consideration of all factors before even a limited judgment can be made. Children, however, generally encounter questions that can be answered unequivocally and thus provide positive reinforcement.

Because of past experiences, adults frequently view a new situation in terms of traditional, cultural, religious, or institutional correctness. Today, for example, we see less rigidity, or greater conflict, as divergent religious and cultural groups have more direct contact.

The third factor concerns the effect of solutions to problems. While a child's answer to a question may provide nothing more than the basis for a grade, an adult's solution to a problem may affect others. Thus adult's solutions tend to be more dramatic in the scope of their effects.

Finally, no general assumption can be made about the expectations of adult learners. Because adults generally are not required by law to attend school, they do not come with the same expectations as children have. The adult, because of work experience and personal background, may hold entirely different views than the adult educator who has set expectations for a given class or course.

Kidd puts forth five concepts as guidelines for the investigation of the key differences among adult learners (Table 3-1).

As stated earlier, most research dealing with learning has focused on children. While there are numerous texts and articles dealing

Table 3-1. Kidd's differentiation between pedagogy and andragogy

Identifying term	Interpretation
Life-span	Various physical, personality, sensory and intellectual changes occur over the years, e.g., variations in sensory capacities.
Maturation	Adults tend to grow toward self-direction, self-discipline, and autonomy, e.g., desire to direct own learning.
Adult experience	Adults have more experiences, differing in kind and organized in different ways, e.g., greater range of experience among adults than among children.
Self-learner	Adults are "inner directed," e.g., learning opportunities are related to individual's need.
Time	Adults perceive time differently, e.g., time may be as valuable as money or effort.

with the "normal" 4 year old, it would be difficult to find much information about the "normal" 35 year old. Kidd's idea of *life-span* involves a consideration of the whole life and the changes that occur which may affect how adults learn. Conducting a safety program in which one expects the learners to move immobilized "patients" from their beds to a point of safety will differentiate many physical abilities among the learners. Some of these may be related to life-span; others may be related to the health status of each individual. At times we have heard "older" nurses say that they are not going to work on the general medical-surgical units because they are "getting too old for all that." Recognition of variations in sensory capacities, physical abilities, personality, and intellectual capabilities assists the staff development educator in facilitating learning.

Maturation recognizes the adult's desire to have self-direction and self-discipline. It

behooves us as staff development educators to study position descriptions to ascertain the parameters placed on the positions and then to relate these limitations to the persons within that category. Once new employees understand what is expected of them, they will likely exercise their maturity and gain individual satisfaction from the position without outside direction. However, we find both extremes—the employees who always want to do everything their own way and those who exercise so much self-discipline within defined limitations that they are not creative, thus losing the sense of autonomy.

Another concept Kidd cites is that of *adult experience*. Because adults have lived longer, they have more experience with which to relate new situations. They also have different kinds of experiences (work, parenthood, etc.) that may interrelate to cause individual differences in perception. Adults also tend to organize their experiences in different ways. Thus when facing a group of eight new employees, it may be found that few commonalities exist or that while all the individuals have had certain general experiences, each has interpreted them in a different way. The knowledge that adults bring certain experiences to a position should be considered by the staff development educator in planning additional experiences for each employee. For example, knowing that an individual has had a recent death in the immediate family should alert the staff development educator to certain reactions this individual may have in working with a terminally ill patient.

Kidd's idea of the *self-learner* involves motivation or that particular moment when an individual wants to learn something because it is crucial. New employees tend to be interested in those skills they do not already possess. They are eager to learn the skills that are expected of them in their new positions. If the principles of a given skill are the same as those previously learned, but the actual procedure differs and the agency is rigid in its expectation of using the defined procedure only, the employee may be willing to relearn an old skill in order to adhere to the system. In continuing education efforts, we are frequently surprised at the number of people who elect to participate in a given offering. Perhaps electrical hazards were discussed four weeks ago and only a handful of employees appeared. Yet now almost all of the personnel from a given unit are present. During the intervening time something may have happened on the unit, such as an electrical fire, that resulted in the personnel's desire to learn more about electrical safety. To be aware of the adult's learning needs and to respond to those needs are two of the primary functions of the staff development educator.

Kidd's final point is one with which staff development educators are particularly familiar. *Time* is a crucial entity. How often have we heard, "I don't have time to go to that class. I have too much to do"? Whether to plan an offering in three one-hour sessions, and hope everyone attends the full series, or to have one three-hour session is a problem with which persons in continuing education contend almost daily. Even in the personal lives of adults, many decisions are based on time rather than cost. Time has become so valuable that each educational effort must be scrutinized closely to be certain it is worth the time and effort. While it is ideal to initiate learning experiences on an individual basis in the clinical area, it is not always practical to do so. Therefore identifying a segment of time when the learners are able to attend is of great significance.

Miller's differentiation[8]

Miller's delineation of differences between adults and children is summarized in Table 3-2.

Adults need or want to learn such a variety of things that it is sometimes difficult to provide group instruction. This variance must be recognized if each learner's needs are to be met. This variance relates to the fact that children tend to be a more homogeneous group, while adults tend to be more *heterogeneous* (see Kidd's concept of life-span). It is difficult to know the starting point when

Table 3-2. Miller's differentiation between pedagogy and andragogy

Identifying term	Interpretation
Heterogeneity	Learners in a group do not have very similar backgrounds, e.g., ethnic, social, and economic variances.
Structure	Previous experiences give individuals certain expectations, e.g., perceptions.
Maturity	Adults respond in more independent ways, e.g., desire to be involved in decisions.

the group has a variety of backgrounds; that is, begin where each learner is. Even in a group that may appear to be homogeneous, such as licensed practical nurses, there is variance. One may have been licensed by waiver, not even required to take a test; another may have completed a formal course, but have no experience, and others may have completed a formal course and have considerable clinical practice. This latter group may differ considerably in how they respond to a specific learning experience because of types of settings, focus of clinical practice, previous policies, reason for current employment, and other factors.

Structure is the second factor Miller cites as a basis for differentiation. This term relates to Kidd's "adult experience" and involves perception—the unique meaning an individual gives a particular experience by virtue of other past experiences. We all know that this factor can work to our advantage or to our disadvantage, depending on past experience. The female worker who had a painful, frightening experience during the birth of her child could have a traumatic experience as an employee in the maternity area. Yet that same person may have had several positive experiences with elderly persons in the community and thus could relate well in a geriatric setting. If we as adult educators do not capitalize on positive past experiences, we may block learning.

The third factor Miller emphasizes is *maturity*. While we all know some children who are more mature than some adults, we generally assume that adults are more mature. Adults do not want forced decisions; they want assistance in identifying problems and alternative solutions. Unfortunately, many of us violate this premise in working with adults. Initially, it is far more expedient to make a decision than to wait for others to decide. However, the time lost in allowing others to participate in a decision is usually more than compensated for in the implementation stage. Because more people are a part of the decision and can voice their own feelings, they are more committed to successful implementation than are those who are told to do something "because that's the decision." Thus while a director of nursing can make a quick decision concerning a new nursing practice, it may never be implemented if the practitioners do not believe it facilitates their care of patients.

Knowles' differentiation[9]

Most recently, Knowles identified his beliefs about adult learners. He cites four major characteristics—self-concept, experience, readiness to learn, and orientation to learning (Table 3-3).

Knowles' *self-concept* relates to Kidd's "maturation" and to Miller's "maturity" and deals with the greater independence of adults. Adults need to be recognized as individuals capable of making their own decisions. Generally, they do not respond favorably to being treated like children and are uncomfortable in typical classroom situations. They want to be respected. When these self-concept needs are ignored and adults are placed in learning situations that do not incorporate their needs, they tend to resist learning. As stated earlier, if such an offering is based on voluntary attendance, they may not appear!

Once again, learning situations should allow for as much participation by the learners as possible. The Chinese philosopher Confucius

Table 3-3. Knowles' differentiation between pedagogy and andragogy

Identifying term	Interpretation
Self-concept	Adults make more of their own decisions about what they will do, what they will buy, and what they will learn, e.g., desire to be involved in decisions.
Experience	The amount and variety of experience provides a broader basis for reacting to new experiences, e.g., perceptions.
Readiness to learn	The motivation connected with a particular learning experience is based on the individual's "need" for that experience, e.g., desire to become "oriented" precedes desire to develop specialized skills.
Orientation to learning	Adults tend to focus on immediate problems, e.g., information to use now that relates to frequently occurring problems is better received.

expresses the ideal learning process—"I hear and I forget, I see and I remember, I do and I understand." Being able to use what has been learned reinforces new knowledge. This is especially true with adults who are more action oriented. If an instructor discusses interviewing techniques, a practice session immediately following allows the adult to exhibit unique alterations of the process due to past experiences and to the self-concept factor.

Experience is particularly significant with regard to adult learners because of the amount and variety. Knowles, citing that children tend to identify themselves in terms of external sources, states that adults differ because they are a culmination of experiences. In the 1960's a popular party game was "Who Am I?" People were asked to think of three statements about themselves; then others tried to guess what the statements were. Frequently used

Table 3-4. Key differentiations between pedagogy and andragogy

Differentiations by authors			Key meaning
KIDD	MILLER	KNOWLES	
Maturation	Maturity	Self-concept	Independency
Adult experience	Structure	Experience	Perceptions
Self-learner		Readiness to learn	Motivation
Time		Orientation to learning	Immediacy, focus, and effort
Life-span	Heterogeneity		Variety of learning needs

statements dealt with occupation, marriage role, parenthood, and hobbies. Experience (Kidd's "adult experience" and Miller's "structure") can affect the learning rate depending on the nature of related, previous experiences. In addition, Knowles points out that adults contribute to each other's learning through sharing information about experiences. How many times have you attended a meeting and said, "I learned so much from the others in my group"? At times the speaker can fail to deliver the message, but the meeting is still worthwhile because of the interaction among the learners. Better use of the learner's experience allows for broader based learning.

The third factor, *readiness to learn,* has particular significance. That "teachable moment" so often escapes the learner and the teacher. Part of the problem lies in the failure to examine the individual's learning needs. For example, Freire found that adults in Brazil learned to read in forty hours *if* the first words they learned were charged with political meaning.[10] He capitalized on their need to understand and take action. Similarly, staff development educators must determine what the learners really need and want to know. A clinical presentation of various decubitus care methods is not useful for the nurse whose immediate concern is with medication side effects. Conversely, the nurse in the clinical setting who has difficulty holding persons accountable eagerly awaits the next class on leadership. It is the responsibility of the staff development educator or clinical expert to capitalize on the "teachable moment"

and to help the nurses deal with their specific problems.

In Knowles' discussion of this particular point (Kidd's "self-learner"), Havinghurst's model of adult life developmental tasks is cited. Should this model be studied, it must be remembered that in a changing society the demarcations cannot be absolute. Hence we find many people in the middle-age group coping with the tasks attributed to those in early adulthood. The important concept to retain is that a particular experience must meet the learner's needs if their readiness to learn is to be capitalized upon.

Knowles' final area of distinction is that of *orientation to learning.* This concept relates to Kidd's "time" differentiation. Knowles' two key factors are topic and time. Adults focus more on problems than on subject matter and desire immediacy of application rather than a reference for the future. Good examples of orientation to problems are the "how to" books that have spanned the horizon of potential problems. Generally these books are not studied as a basis for future action. Rather they are grabbed as the basement fills with water, as the garden withers, or as the children threaten to leave home. Kidd's use of time, however, relates more to its value than to its immediacy of effect.

• • •

Table 3-4 summarizes the key differentiations cited by the three authors. It is not intended to be absolute or all encompassing. Rather its purpose is to provide a brief conceptual outline of the key points of three adult educators.

IMPLICATIONS FOR STAFF DEVELOPMENT EDUCATORS

So what does all this mean? As Knowles points out, the andragogical approach is more concerned with the process than with the content. To understand some of the significant points about the differences in adult education, we need to refer to the staff development process (Fig. 1-2).

The three key factors, input, process, and output, are affected by the characteristics of adult learners. It is understood that this same process could be used with a pedagogical approach but various segments would be significantly different because of the differences that exist between adults and children.

Input

Seven broad areas of input have been identified for the purposes of staff development. Although standards of care may be developed within an agency, we frequently find that the agency has not made these standards explicit. Rather extra-agency standards are accepted as the norm. For example, nurses may wish to refer to *Standards for Nursing Services*[11] or to the standards issued by Medicare, the Joint Commission on Accreditation of Hospitals, and the state licensure board and health department. The overall goals that reflect an agency's purpose and its view of health care help to define role expectations for the various positions within the agency.

Establishing goals, standards, and role expectations that are consistent with the philosophy of the agency, the nursing service, and staff development provides a basis for the first phase of meeting adults' learning needs. Knowing what is expected or required provides the foundation for identifying the individual's learning needs. Although this important aspect is discussed in depth in Chapter 7, the issue must be included here. Examining the learner's knowledge and skills in relation to the expectations or requirements helps the staff develop-

ment educator identify the learner's particular discrepancies. While these discrepancies may be clear to the educator, they may not be so to the learner. The learner must be motivated to change his pattern of behavior. For some, the motivation may be the result of factors such as economy and prestige. Others, however, may be motivated to become a "better practitioner." Whatever the motivational reason, the staff development educator's responsibility is to identify the discrepancies between the learner's ability and the expectations of him. The learners must be involved in the identification of these discrepancies. Helping the learners to identify for themselves what the discrepancies are facilitates learners' internalizing the need for change. Only after each learner's profile is established do the learning needs become more evident.

Adults, as self-directed people, need to be involved in the decisions that affect them. Due to the nature of certain previous experiences, it is sometimes difficult for the individual to recognize a discrepancy. For example, a nurse with several years of experience in an operating room may resent an intensive orientation to a new operating room. However, this orientation may be justified if the role expectations or the types of operative cases differ greatly from the other agency.

Thus in the input stage the learners need to know what the expectations are; they need to be aware of their current knowledge and skills; they need to be involved in defining their needs; they need to have previous experience recognized; and they need to be recognized as individuals.

Process

The process stage occurs within the framework of the existing planning mechanism and involves climate setting. The climate that the learners enter may alter their attitudes toward participation in staff development. It is important to capitalize on establishing an informal atmosphere, allowing for discussion, and recognizing each learner as an individual.

As much as possible, objectives of specific

activities should be behaviorally oriented and demonstrable in the clinical setting. Although this is not always feasible, it should be remembered that the adult is concerned with the time element as much as with the effort. If a segment of time is spent discussing or practicing some particular nursing skill, learners need to see the impact in the clinical area (or a simulated clinical area). Without this reinforcement they may "forget" the skill or adapt it in ways that do not meet acceptable standards.

One important aspect that should be considered in the process stage is the group size. Borman,[12] for example, believes the most effective group size to be from five to seven persons. He states that a group of ten or more is too large to allow for adequate discussion. A group with fewer than five is frequently too narrow in scope and too limited. In the small groups, everyone usually talks with everyone else, while in the larger groups, individuals tend to speak only to those they recognize as group leaders or not at all. At times the larger groups seems to become a smaller one because a few of the members carry on the discussion as if the others were not there. Thus, with regard to adult learning, the size of the group is of major importance. Eugene Peckham, of Western Training Services in Long Beach, California, has devised a formula for the effectiveness of group size. His *group effectiveness quotient,* based on the fact that we communicate most effectively on a one-to-one basis (a two-group), is as follows:

$$P = \frac{N(N - 1)}{2}$$

In the equation, P represents pairs, the possible number of two-groups, while N represents the number in the group. The greater the number of two-groups, the more chance there is for misunderstanding. Because adults gain additional benefits from small-group work, the instructor may want to consider reinforcing lectures with small-group work or individualized follow-up discussions. Peckham (personal correspondence, 1973) adds, "A co-

hesive group—one in which production, synergy, and communicative efficiency are high—requires at least 50% of its two-groups working. This furnishes the leader the goal of getting 51% of his participants 'warmed-up'—capable of productive contributions, of engaging in instrumental dialogues."

A variety of teaching methods are based on the concepts of andragogy. These are discussed in depth in Chapter 9.

Finally, in implementing and evaluating the program, one needs to be aware of individual differences. If speed is essential to the acceptable performance of a skill, the time limitation should be spelled out in the objectives. Thus individuals will know what criteria they are to be measured against. If the evaluation is to be done in the clinical area, then this fact should be clearly stated to the learners. Part of a feeling of trust develops when one knows how he will be judged.

In order to be realistic in implementing a given program, the individual differences of the learners should be considered. As cited earlier, while the repetition of experience may be frustrating for a new employee, it may be essential. Striking a happy medium in which the individual can gain the necessary additional experience without feeling frustrated is a difficult but necessary task.

In implementing a program, an attempt should be made to allow as much self-direction by the learner as possible. For example, the desired outcome may require that the new employees know the nursing practice policies related to the clinical area: some learners may want to study the policy manual; others may want to review it briefly then observe in the clinical area; and still others may wish to compare the policies with those of the previous employing agency and discuss areas of difference. Although the learners have taken different paths to reach the same goal, they should be able to cite the policies that relate to their clinical areas.

Another key concept to remember is that adults tend to have different perceptions of a situation. While this factor may prove favorable, it may also be disadvantageous. For example, most of us in hospital settings would have similar perceptions when reading an order stating "CVP q1h." Immediately we would know that the central venous pressure is to be recorded hourly. Thus, depending on the learners, it might not be necessary in an orientation to discuss the terminology and purpose in depth. However, it may be that some of the learners have not previously performed the procedure in a manner that meets the current expectations. Thus the perception these individuals have may work to their disadvantage. It would be necessary to reorient these learners so that they perform a familiar procedure in a new way. Generally, many agencies do not adhere strictly to defined step-by-step procedures that must be executed. However, all agencies expect a procedure to be performed in a safe manner that will achieve accurate and desirable end results.

Output

Performance behaviors may be as varied as the number of individuals in the group. Although there should be a range of flexibility in the achievement of expected outcomes, there are certain criteria that must be met before an individual can be identified as having met the expectation. Agencies that have rigid expectations may have very frustrated employees who feel that they are unable to function as adults. However, agencies that have very relaxed expectations (or none defined) will also have frustrated employees, because they will not know how to function.

Thus it is necessary for an agency to have stated nursing practice policies and certain procedures for implementing these policies in a uniform manner. As described in Chapter 5, policies are broad statements giving direction to behavior or functioning. A procedure then describes "how to" behave or perform a function according to agency expectations. Learners need to be aware of the procedures and how each is enforced before they are comfortable in their own behavior. In situations where the explicit policy differs from the

implied, there may be erratic behavior or adherence to the method most accepted by the employee peer group. It is imperative that the staff development educator recognizes these impinging factors in observing behavior.

STATEMENTS OF ADULT CHARACTERISTICS
Adult learning

While it is not necessary to enumerate the differences of adult learners, it may be advantageous to incorporate into the philosophy of staff development a statement concerning adult learning and its significance within the agency.

Research has shown that adults in an employment situation do not learn in the same way as children. Therefore it is important for staff development educators to be aware of these differences. The following five statements might be made regarding the adult learner.

1. *Adults must want to learn and must feel the need for a particular knowledge or skill.* Adults want to learn something that will help them in the everyday work situation. Unless they have an inner motivation and feel the need to learn, there will be little benefit from their attendance at staff development activities. Preparation of the employee for staff development activities, entailing counseling and identification of the needs for a specific skill or knowledge, is important to the success of the subsequent learning process.

2. *Adults prefer learning based on active involvement and the problems they face in the working environment.* They want the chance to use what they have learned before they forget it; therefore practical experience in conjunction with formal classes is important for the retention of new knowledge or skills. A relationship between the subject matter and the everyday work situation is vital to adult learning. Adult learners prefer to start with their own specific problems, work out the solution, and then examine how the theory applies. They resist a straight presentation of theory that is representative of the "school approach."

3. *The opportunity to question and the freedom to disagree in an environment that allows for mature relationships facilitate adult learning.* The adult comes to class with many life experiences that influence his perception of the learning task. The learner needs the opportunity to present personal views in an accepting atmosphere that is conducive to them. This kind of give-and-take also provides the teacher with some idea of the learner's acquired knowledge.

4. *Adults want guidance and to know how they are progressing.* Adults tend to resist competition such as grades and tests and to withdraw from learning situations that are potentially humiliating. They need to know on an individual basis of their progress in learning. This can best be accomplished by involving each learner in self-evaluation along with a teacher evaluation.

5. *An informal setting facilitates adult learning.* An environment conducive to relaxation (ventilated rooms, appropriate seating arrangement, etc.) is desirable. Reducing the resemblance to a schoolroom atmosphere increases the possibility that learning will occur. Therefore conference-type settings are recommended when possible.

SUMMARY

Briefly, an understanding of adult learning is important for the planning as well as the implementation of the staff development process. The outcome will be affected by the application of andragogical concepts. Although it is not always necessary to make explicit statements about a given group of learners, one should be aware of individual differences as well as general group differences before planning a program, in conducting it, and in expecting output. Knowing the learners gives direction to the educator's role.

REFERENCES

1. Teaching adults is different . . . or is it? In Techniques for teachers of adults, Washington, D. C., no date, National Association for Public Continuing and Adult Education.
2. Toffler, A.: Future shock, New York, 1970, Random House, Inc.
3. Stein, L. S.: Adult learning principles: The individual curriculum and nursing leadership, J. Cont. Educ. Nurs. 2(6):7, 1971.
4. Mead, M.: Thinking ahead: why is education obsolete? Harvard Bus. Rev. 36(6):23, 1958.
5. Thorndike, E. L., et al.: Adult learning, New York, 1928, Macmillan Publishing Co., Inc.
6. Powell, J. W.: Learning comes of age, New York, 1956, Association Press.
7. Kidd, J. R.: How adults learn, New York, 1959, Association Press.
8. Miller, H. L.: Teaching and learning in adult education, New York, 1964, Macmillan Publishing Co., Inc.
9. Knowles, M.: The modern practice of adult education, New York, 1970, Association Press.
10. Illich, I.: Why we must abolish schooling, N. Y. Rev. Books 15(1):9, 1970.
11. American Nurses' Association: Standards for nursing services, Kansas City, Mo., 1973, The Association.
12. Borman, E. G.: Discussion and group methods: theory and practice, New York, 1969, Harper & Row, Publishers.

BIBLIOGRAPHY

Brunner, E. de S., Wilder, D. S., Kirchner, C., and Newberry, J. S., Jr.: An overview of adult education research, Chicago, 1959, Adult Education Association of the U. S. A.

Dill, W., Crowston, W. B. S., and Elton, E. J.: Strategies for self-education, Harvard Bus. Rev. 43(6):119, 1965.

Ingalls, J. D., and Arceri, J. M.: A trainer's guide to andragogy, Washington, D. C., 1972, Department of Health, Education, and Welfare.

Knowles, M. S.: Gearing adult education for the seventies, J. Cont. Educ. Nurs. 1(1):11, 1970.

Lorge, I.: The adult learner. In Psychology of adults, Washington, D. C., 1963, Adult Education Association.

New Jersey State Department of Education: The teaching of adults, Trenton, no date, Bureau of Adult Education.

Ohliger, J., and McCarthy, C.: Lifelong learning or lifelong schooling? Syracuse, 1971, ERIC Clearinghouse on Adult Education.

Stein, L. S.: Adult learning principles, the individual curriculum and nursing leadership. J. Cont. Educ. Nurs. 2(6):7, 1971.

This, L. E., and Lippitt, G. L.: Learning theories and training, Washington, D. C., no date, Leadership Resources, Inc.

4 Motivation and staff development

DRUSILLA POOLE

You cannot teach a man anything; you can only help him to find it within himself.

GALILEO

How to reconcile the personal goals of staff members with the demands of their professional situations—such is the problem of motivation.

Concern with the subject of motivation on the part of nursing administrators indicates the frequent failure to elicit participation and to effect change through staff development efforts. This concern with motivation may lead nurses to look for more effective motivators within staff development. Problems in motivation are not peculiar to nursing or even to the health professions. Throughout the country in all kinds of workshops and conferences for the varied disciplines, motivation looms great in importance whenever groups come to grips with the subject of staff development, the needs for improvement of practice, and the problems encountered by administrative and educational leaders.

Webster's dictionary says that *to motivate* is "to provide with a motive" or to "impel" or "incite." Motivation has its origin and residence within the self, so that acting in accord with a motive may be regarded as self-expression. All motivation should arise from a genuine interest in the present activity or what it leads to.[1] Thus motivation is that *within* the individual, rather than without, which incites him to act. It is an emotion or desire, a want if conscious, operating on one's will and serving as an impetus to action. In personnel management it is sometimes neces-sary to find the means with which to motivate a staff member to take a specific action in order to satisfy a specific need. At the core of motivation in this context is that behind every act, movement, or thought lies the question of utility to the individual. This factor of utility to the person provides insight into the great variations that are possible in individual adjustment. A person's actual motives in behavior may be quite different from his stated intentions, because the expectations and acceptance of others enter in. At any rate the basic motivation for all individuals is the desire for ego satisfaction via acceptable and useful channels or via unsatisfactory adjustment (this is in terms of the individual's satisfaction and not the approval of others). Such explanations are necessarily relevant to motivation, because one is prone to label lagging members of a group as "lacking motivation." Actually, motivation is a quantitative driving force. The "lazy tramps" or the "deadwood" may be just as strongly motivated to be what they are as is the highly successful executive of the firm. They use different means and seek different goals, but they may be just as satisfied and adjusted. There is general agreement that motives are internal factors that arouse, direct, and integrate a person's behavior. Motives are not observed directly but are inferred from behavior and assumed to exist in order to explain behavior.[2]

Other individuals are influenced by *their*

desires and not *ours*, for there exist within all persons certain "springs of action" that make them think, believe, or act. Their "springs of action" must be reached if we are to influence their behavior. Usually we reach others through a combination of the following: (1) reason, the capacity to think and to use basic intelligence and knowledge; (2) rationalization or pretense that there is a logical reason for doing what the person wants to do or has done; and (3) emotions or feelings in relation to satisfaction of basic human needs. A word of warning here! Remember that *man is not a creature of reason*. Attempts at changing the smoking habits of people through publicity about the danger of cancer have demonstrated the ineffectiveness of appealing to reason. It would seem that the other two avenues, involving the desires, are the ones that provide the motive power for what man does. Therefore if we are to influence others, we must discover these desires, harness them, and then use them as motivators. Remember that the same water that floods can turn turbines!

HIERARCHY OF MOTIVES

Maslow's theory of a hierarchy of motives states that a person's needs are satisfied from lower to higher levels of priority.[3] These basic needs or goals are arranged in a structure of prepotency suggesting that at a given moment the most prepotent goal will monopolize consciousness and utilize all energies and capacities of the individual. This structure from low to high includes physiological needs, safety needs, the needs to belong and be loved, esteem needs, and the need for self-actualization. Man's ultimate response is self-fulfillment according to what he is potentially capable of becoming and involves what Maslow terms "growth motivation." Man's capacity for creation and aesthetic response seems to be delayed, denied, and forgotten until lower order needs are satisfied. Man's ultimate motive power is the sense of value and the sense of importance. This sense of values imposes on life incredible labors.[1]

Physiological needs include those that are life-sustaining, self-preserving, and essential to the comfort or equilibrium of human beings. The prominence of these needs has been unquestionably established, but it is sometimes ignored (for instance, when educators or administrators try to motivate a person who has had no sleep to learn or to participate in some new, complex situation).

Safety and security are also recognized as basic human needs. Although money and economic comfort are closely associated with security, safety represents man's desire to be physically and psychologically secure. A person in a subordinate position has the need to depend on the decisions and judgments of supervisors. He needs to know what to expect in the way of consistent and fair relationships. Security is learned through the consistency of discipline and order. To be a good driver and to find driving an automobile a relaxed and pleasant pastime, a person must feel security in the consistency of signals, laws, the fairness of law enforcement personnel, and the conformity on the part of fellow drivers to certain rules of behavior. Man does seek consistency and equilibrium, but he also seems to take pleasure in upsetting things. "He seems most vigorously human when he deliberately precipitates himself into just manageable difficulties, then works to restore order."[4] Human nature is too complex and exciting to fit neatly into any formulated structure that lacks extensive interpretation and patterning of the choices or channels open to man. The desire for new experiences, those exploratory excursions on the path of purposeful and pleasant change, is a motivator. It can incite an individual to revolt against sameness and monotony or to embrace the excitement of learning and behaving in a new way. Boredom is defined as the lack or deprivation of stimuli. A curiosity motive (a search for stimuli) plays a role in exploration, discovery, and learning.[2] Man is completely dependent on continuous sensory input from the environment, but he is also physically in need of variations in that input to maintain the healthy level of sensitivity that keeps him most appropriately in touch with his world. It is difficult to define curiosity and exploration merely as changes in stimuli, because all behavioral response is a change in itself. In accepting a curiosity motive, we recognize an intrinsic drive that appears to have its own purpose.[5]

The *needs for love and belonging* focus on man's relating and reacting to others. The need for social activity and human stimulation is a qualitative one, but most individuals desire affectionate relationships with people and a respected place in the group. Acceptance and approval by one's peer group are prime motivators in behavior. They must be recognized and utilized by those who would influence behavior and be evaluated as deterrents or expediters in staff development. They explain the lack of motivation to think or to behave differently from one's group or peers. The desire to be understood and appreciated is man's bid for acceptance. He wants to express himself in terms of his virtues, limitations, and problems without censure. He seeks out those who respond to him as an individual and whose empathetic reply reflects neither blame nor shock. Educators and administrators learn that acceptance, both verbal and nonverbal, affects relationships dramatically and influences motivation (example of cohesive groups).

Esteem or recognition is one of the basic human needs and is thought of as the desire for power and property. At times the overemphasis on rank, salary, and promotion indicates a narrowed concept of the meaning of esteem. A person wants to feel worthwhile as an individual and in what he produces. Appreciation and praise from a supervisor may assist in this. Acquiring a leadership position and a reputation of note is important to an individual's sense of worth, but while the basic need is constant, the means by which it is expressed often vary. Such diversity in means may be illustrated by the behaviors of a group of individuals in which one will have the neatest uniform, one will break the most rules, one will outdrink the others, one will know the most gossip, and another will collect degrees. Acceptance of self, the development of a self-concept, and a feeling of personal worth relate to behavioral motives. Man desires to maintain or establish a positive image of the self. This operates as a powerful motive and helps to explain why people are able to sustain themselves with pride. If we accept an innate social drive, to threaten a man's self-esteem is to threaten his belief that he is a worthwhile person with a position of dignity in the society.[2] Problems in individual behavior may stem from an inability to accept the self, denial of certain aspects of the self, and a person's failure to emerge as an autonomous and unique individual. This self-concept is significant in motivation, but caution must be exercised in its use as a motivating factor. Frustration of an individual often results from a conflict between motivation and an apperception of self-inadequacy. Although an individual's own self-concept is the key to behavior, it is constantly undergoing modifications in relation to inner tensions, concepts of reality, and changes in emotionality with age and social experiences. Thus inherent in the individual are mechanisms for effecting normal adjustment and control. Identification, projection, and formation of ego ideals enhance his self-concept when other psychological maneuvers leave him quite dissatisfied. In considering techniques of motivation, one realizes that by working through an individual's self-concept, the "self" is made to act as an instrument for change in behavior. The self becomes the creator of supportive relationships and the instigator of corrective maneuvers in its behavior patterns.

CLIMATE FOR MOTIVATION

Climate for motivation denotes the administrative and educational environment in which one works. The term "climate" refers to a potential for both comfort and growth. Before the proper climate can be determined, those things that interfere with or make possible a realization of the needs of the staff must be identified. Approval, the knowledge that the nursing administration will support sound decisions, is one key to a good climate. Strictness of discipline and enforced standards of performance have no adverse effect on climate if workers have confidence in those who enforce discipline. Communication is basic to approval, and language is basic to communication. A bad climate may result if the administration is speaking the "language of productivity and efficiency" when the personnel have a need to hear the "language of motivation."

Administrators and educators must make an attempt to be heard and to be understood. They must identify and reinforce appropriate actions that reflect the needs of personnel, because the meeting of these needs (job satisfaction) is their motivating force and their language. Not until staff development programs are put into the language of motivation will a staff hear what is being said or be motivated toward ego involvement. We believe that supervision in the nursing setting must concern itself with the climate for learning, because a staff of professional personnel, committed to their professional responsibilities, must be in the learning business. When job satisfaction is viewed as an end in itself, complacency and a self-contained "all's well" philosophy often result.[6] A healthy discontent with current performance can create a climate conducive to learning. The highly satisfied workers are not necessarily the most productive workers. Job satisfaction is the *result* of performance behavior rather than the cause. High and low performers differ in their perceptions of the rewards to be derived from a job through expression of autonomy and self-realization.[7] These are the satisfactions that motivate. The motivation seekers are most often inner-directed and self-sufficient persons whose achievement of personal goals is not facilitated by management actions that overrate maintenance needs, but rather by actions that provide conditions for motivation.[8]

The motivation-maintenance theory, based on Herzberg's study of factors in the work set-ting, has important implications for staff development.[9] Herzberg's study supported the existence of distinct and separate "satisfiers" in the work setting that serve as motivators and promote growth. The attainment of happiness requires psychological growth through job enrichment that constitutes a continuous management function. His definition of "satisfiers" (motivation factors) identifies the strong determinants of job satisfaction—achievement, recognition, the work itself, and responsibility in terms of advancement. However, these factors are applicable only if work is meaningful to the worker. By contrast, the "dissatisfiers" (hygiene or maintenance factors) reflect the preventive and environmental atmosphere of the setting—company policy and administration, supervision, salary, interpersonal relations, and working conditions. Maintenance factors may prevent discontent with the job but do not lead the individual to any significant psychological growth. Attending to hygiene needs is important, but effects of improved hygiene last only a short time and the needs are recurrent. Herzberg's strongest indictment is against "hygiene seekers" in key positions who determine the atmosphere of the unit and demand that their own motivational characteristics be instilled in their subordinates. Such supervisors cannot help having an adverse effect on staff development, which should be aimed at the personal growth and self-actualization of the staff members.[10] Staff development programs should be geared to the motivation of personnel within the work setting. Three goals of such programs would be (1) a change in emphasis from hygiene to self-fulfillment that will hopefully develop loyalty to the unit or work force, (2) job enlargement with the aim of opening up new areas for psychological growth, and (3) education to prevent technological obsolescence, poor performance, and administrative failure.[10]

Some problems in motivation stem from the very narrowed concepts of staff development held by many nursing personnel. The impact of these "conceptual handicaps" plagues both those who are responsible for staff development programs and those who would make staff development an integral part of supervision and the work style of nursing personnel.[11] One stifling definition of staff development held by nurses is that it is a formal classroom-type instruction or a "monthly meeting"; if defined simply as *personal and professional growth*, problems of motivation within staff development would be greatly reduced. Much effort is needed to clear up all the misconceptions about education and academic programs and their relationships to nursing and nursing services. Perhaps many of the problems in motivation are caused by confusion in the minds of personnel about the utilization and the value of the educative process.

Related to these problems in conceptualization is the caliber of individuals on whom nursing groups depend for leadership in staff development. Problems in staff motivation result when leaders are inadequately prepared in psychology, sociology, adult education, and group and conference skills. Such leadership cannot effect maximum in-service growth for their personnel. Leaders must be able to evaluate motivational problems, be proficient in handling these problems, and approach individuals in such a manner as to avoid unnecessary resistance. If the group leader views the learning activities as worthwhile and important enough for full-scale endorsement, this attitude can contribute notably to a learner's interest and enthusiasm. The leader who demonstrates faith in the program to be presented and in the staff's ability to assimilate new knowledge will very likely be able to solve any problems in motivation. The wise leader will make no pledges about attaining educational goals but promises only to assist the group members in constantly appraising the work being done and the progress toward *their* stated goals. Qualified leadership is needed to ensure the high caliber of nursing practice and the retention of qualified practitioners to which the profession is commited.

The "important others" with whom individuals work directly influence their motivation, as do the group setting and the social structure in which they live and work. The "important others" are those with whom a person participates in the performance of his role and with whom he shares common values. The group places a positive valuation on the person, for the group or "social circle" needs the individual's cooperation for the realization of its goals and maintenance of its established and accepted values.[12] Pace and participation are determined to a large extent by the degree to which individuals are willing to become ego-involved and by the investment they consider worthwhile to make in education. Being involved with a group that has a particular goal will result in motivation to participate actively and to be more aggressive than if the group has little direction. Individual differences in sensitivity to and in awareness of needs are basic to the degree of willingness to become involved and of belief in the importance of that involvement.

The results of any program should be measured in terms of what happens to the group when individuals decide to act, to stick to their convictions, and to make their own decisions about learning. Comprehensive and meaningful goals must be accomplished one step at a time, with some reward through recognition and status for all the participating group members.

CONCEPT OF CHANGE

Because it brings about change, progress in staff development may precipitate resistance. There are many logical reasons why people resist change. People dislike being in ambiguous situations; they like to know where they stand and what is going on. If they do not see the necessity or reason behind it, they cannot understand why change should be effected. Because it implies criticism of present practice, change may represent a threat and an indictment that evokes defensiveness. Change often dictates that a person become so different from the peer group that it would mean severing ties with fellow workers and establishing new and strange relationships within the familiar setting. A central sociological assumption about motivation is that a person tends to engage in actions that help to maintain the valuation received from associates at or above a given level. Acceptance of change may need to be postponed in order that the person ascertain the opinions of the reference group. Not all of an individual's associates have the same relevance with regard to the maintenance of favorable evaluation and continuing acceptance.[13] If the change alters an individual's position in the group, threatens esteem received from peers, and deviates from values set by the group, then it becomes a threat to his personal goals. A person is more comfortable in not doing what is asked if group feeling runs against the request. The freedom to deviate seems to be proportionate to the degree to which the individual feels accepted by the group. The less secure we are about group membership, the more strictly we need to adhere to opinions, norms, and goals of the group. On the other hand, those occupying positions of leadership are freer to deviate and should initiate change when it is in the best interests of the group.[14] Quantitatively and qualitatively, resistance is determined in large measure by the individual's position within the group and the security of that position.

How does one deal with resistance to change, which is an obstacle in motivation? The leader must consider that resistance denotes that those involved have some investment in the status quo. First, it is necessary to establish a climate in which people may air their feelings about change. Let the staff know that it is all right for them to have opinions and to verbalize their feelings and fears. Second, allow the whole group to participate in effecting the change. This may be accomplished through discussions regarding current situations, potentialities for change, and the personal stake of those most concerned with proposed innovations. Third, allow for reaction time. This is usually referred to as letting a group "live with an idea for a while." Initial rejection quite often is followed by favorable response. Planning for reaction time is one of the most effective techniques that a leader can employ in getting cooperation and support for proposed change.

Another approach to handling resistance is the process of persuasion. The proposed action should be communicated in a manner that helps the worker visualize the potential satisfaction to be drived from it. Thus a bridge is provided between the proposal of a change and the acceptance of it. This seems a valid answer to the problem of motivating people, for we know two ways of getting people to do what we want them to do—by persuasion and by force. In staff development the concern is for the kind of motivation for learning and for change that is dependent on the participation of individuals in their own development. For this kind of growth, staff development educators, as change agents, must rely on persuasive powers and on the skillful application of motivation techniques geared to the individual's drives and desires.

As a result of continued study and research, a number of interesting ideas have been formulated about motivating factors. For example, negative feedback is more effective than no feedback at all. Learners may be motivated by test results and by constructive criticisms of their performance. The ability to accept and to improve one's self requires some degree of insight into one's potentials and limitations. Learning can, however, be retarded if motivating conditions are too intense; it continues to be wise counsel to say, "Handle motivation factors with care." For those who attempt to modify the behavior of others, as through staff development and counseling, different procedures are indicated if learning occurs through increased tensions rather than tension reduction. The learning situation can be an exciting one and may be most effective when stimulation is strong enough for maximum reinforcement but not strong enough to be disruptive or destructive.[15]

We have learned that motivation in a learning setting is dependent on an individual's needs to defend or to expand the ego and that effectiveness of motivators and reactions to failure vary widely among learners. In spite of all that is known about motivation, the relationship between learning and motivation is not completely understood, but it is generally believed that a learner must be motivated to play an active role before learning can take place.

REFERENCES

1. Brubacher, J. S.: Eclectic philosophy of education, Englewood Cliffs, N. J., 1951, Prentice-Hall, Inc.
2. Murray, E. J.: Motivation and emotion, Englewood Cliffs, N. J., 1964, Prentice-Hall, Inc.
3. Maslow, A. H.: Motivation and personality, New York, 1970, Harper & Row, Publishers.
4. Wrenn, C. G.: The counselor in a changing world, Washington, D. C., 1962, American Personnel and Guidance Association.
5. Fowler, H.: Curiosity and exploratory behavior, New York, 1965, Macmillan Publishing Co., Inc.
6. Hall, B. H.: Creating a climate for learning, Nurs. Outlook 7:422, 1959.
7. Porter, L. W., and Lawler, E. E., III: What job attitudes tell about motivation, Harvard Bus. Rev. 46(1):120, 1968.
8. Myers, M. S.: Who are your motivated workers? Harvard Bus. Rev. 42(1):76, 1964.
9. Herzberg, F., et al.: The motivation to work, New York, 1959, John Wiley & Sons, Inc.
10. Herzberg, F.: Work and the nature of man, New York, 1966, World Publishing Co.
11. Miller, M. A.: Inservice education. I. Conceptual handicaps, Nurs. Outlook 10:691, 1962.
12. Znaniecki, F.: The social role of the man of knowledge, New York, 1940, Columbia University Press.
13. Zetterberg, H. L.: Social theory and social practice, Towata, N. J., 1962, The Bedminster Press, Inc.
14. Cartwright, D., and Lippitt, R.: Group dynamics and the individual. In Bennis, W. G., Benne, D., and Chin, R., editors: The planning of change, New York, 1961, Holt, Rinehart & Winston, Inc.
15. Leuba, C.: Toward some integration of learning theories: the concept of optimal stimulation, Psychol. Rep. 1(1):32, 1955.

BIBLIOGRAPHY

Bennis, W. G., Benne, K. D., and Chin, R.: The planning of change, ed. 2, New York, 1969, Holt, Rinehart & Winston, Inc.

Herzberg, F.: One more time: how do you motivate employees? Harvard Bus. Rev. 46(1):53, 1968.

Lysaught, J.: No carrots, no sticks: motivation in nursing, J. Nurs. Admin. 2(5):43, 1972.

McGregor, D.: The human side of enterprise, New York, 1960, McGraw-Hill Book Co.

Paul, W. J., Jr., Robertson, K. B., and Herzberg, F.: Job enrichment pays off, Harvard Bus. Rev. 47(2):72, 1969.

5 Organization and administration

Well begun is half done.

HORACE

Change permeates today's nursing care delivery systems. The rapidity of change fosters recognition of staff development as a motivating force for planned change and demands that the agency make staff development explicit in the organizational structure.

The impact of new technology and the increased sophistication of nursing science emphasize the need for continued learning. The complexity of human relationships in a society with changing values and life-styles requires development of new leadership styles. Consumers of health care, becoming more knowledgeable about services and costs. want quality at a reasonable cost; this factor is compounded by a changing attitude toward health care. These changes, which add to the complexity of health care, give rise to the need for skilled manpower and for the development of all employees to their highest level of competency.

The concept of staff development for all departments within hospitals is made explicit in the standards of the Joint Commission for Accreditation of Hospitals.[1] Staff development in nursing is cited in the American Nurses' Association's *Standards for Nursing Services.*[2] In seeking approaches to meet the challenges and expectations, it becomes essential that nursing administrators be committed to staff development and to utilize it to support planned change with the goal of improving the nursing care delivery system. Sound and comprehensive planning is a prerequisite of desired change and continued progress.

A statement of the overall staff development philosophy, purpose, and broad goals provides the base for the design of an organizational structure and methodology that will support efforts for the attainment of the goals. Planning encompasses an orientation to the future as well as to the present and includes a design of the overall structure, the determination of the major components, the identification of human and other resources, the formulation of policies and procedures, the design of a system of records and reports, and the delineation of the financial mechanism. All of these factors are interrelated and affect the organization of staff development.

DESIGN OF THE OVERALL STRUCTURE

The aim in initial planning is to establish a data base defining the current status of the agency and what it expects its status to be in the future, taking into account external as well as internal forces, for example, the influence of third-party payers (external) and the number and types of personnel (internal). From an analysis of the data, it can be determined if the present organizational structure can best effect the desired change or if reorganization is necessary. In general the purpose of staff development is to increase the effectiveness and efficiency of the personnel's performance behaviors for the consumers' benefit.

To view the present and project for the future, a data base of the characteristics and factors that can give direction to the design for staff development may be obtained from responses to questions such as the following:

What program is presently offered? Who attends? Are there any coordinated efforts? Should the present program be expanded or diversified?

> For example, if orientation is the only component and is offered on a centralized basis to all employees, what should be provided in the various areas needs to be identified.

Is there coordination or a liaison relationship with an outside agency? Are personnel permitted to attend outside programs? If so, is participation restricted?

> For example, nurses may attend a leadership program outside the agency on a regular basis. The agency may provide opportunities for formal or continuing education for personnel through its affiliation with an educational institution.

What are the human and other resources available? What are the constraints?

> For example, if the agency has limited resources, it might be necessary to have centralized planning and programming.

What are the nursing care programs? Are there special care services such as hemodialysis or coronary care? What skills are necessary to meet the nursing care requirements? What generalizations could be made about the patient population in terms of age groups, acuteness of illness, culture, etc.?

> For example, if a wide range of practice skills is needed by nursing personnel to meet the nursing care requirements, and this is coupled with a high attrition rate among the staff nurse group, it will be evident that frequent and diverse programming may be necessary.

Decisions based on this data should lead first to the design of the "ideal" organizational structure. While the ideal may not be feasible at this point, it will serve as an illustrative model for future efforts. Without this step complacency may develop with regard to the current efforts.

Recognizing the strengths and weaknesses of the agency leads to the formulation of alternative organizational structures.

After weighing the pros and cons, a plan should be selected from the alternatives that will meet the established goals to the greatest degree; based on the economic and personnel constraints, the design selected should meet the critical needs plus priorities of the additional ones.

The next step in the planning process is implementation of the new structure or reorganization of the old. A written plan that guides the agency through required phases over a period of time is helpful. Such a plan also can provide an operational framework for programming. For example, if the outpatient services are to be expanded, this may have implications for the kinds of learning offerings planned. Proposed knowledge of this change allows for the development of necessary programming prior to the advent of the change.

To determine if the essential policy statements or mechanisms for successful implementation are present, another data base for decisions needs to be acquired. Questions now asked include the following:

What statement of policy is necessary to support the new or changed functions?

> For example, if the agency decides that all employees are to attend certain programs or that participation in selected offerings will be based on meeting certain criteria, then a statement of policy should provide that information.

Is realignment or reassignment of responsibilities and resources required?

> For example, annual and long-term budgeting changes may be necessary to channel resources as outlined in the plan.

Has responsibility, authority, and accountability been determined?

> For example, to effect a major change, responsibility and authority should be assigned so that progress or lack of progress can be pinpointed.

At this point information about the new or redesigned organizational structure needs to be communicated and the necessary support systems developed. For example, a communications network needs to be established, and an agreement for the support of the new or changed functions must be reached with the appropriate personnel.

During the initial phases of implementation, a process for periodic review of the new or redesigned organizational structure needs to be defined in order to evaluate the change. Identification of any problems or factors that might indicate that future plans should be changed or modified is an integral part of the process. A review, at least annually, of the long-range plans can be beneficial in terms of projecting farther into the future.

During the planning phase, the responsibility for providing leadership lies with the nursing administration. Nurses who can provide a combination of experience, skills, and knowledge for sound planning should be involved. In a given situation such nurses might include, in addition to the director of nursing, the educator administratively responsible for staff development, other staff development educators, and staff nurses and head nurses. One criterion for selection of nurses in the latter group should be a demonstrated interest in staff development efforts. The interests and skills of these nurses can be utilized not only in designing the organizational structure but also in identifying the specific learning offerings needed to meet the goals and in evaluating the results. Being involved in the planning process can stimulate them to influence change and to take action on decisions they helped make.

CONCEPT OF CENTRALIZATION AND DECENTRALIZATION

Each agency must decide to what extent it will centralize or decentralize its organizational structure. Because organizational structure should emanate from the philosophy of the agency, direction for centralization-decentralization should be found in the philosophy. The concepts of organizational centralization and decentralization express the degree of concentration or dispersion of specific leadership activities.

Centralized approach

The centralized approach to programming is utilized in many nursing services. In this approach a centralized unit sets the pace and assumes the leadership position. Many administrators consider this approach to be the most efficient, effective, and economical. Learning offerings in this approach consist of the presentation of content that relates to the common learning needs of the participants. Because observation of employee performance following participation in a learning offering is one way of evaluating the teaching-learning process, it behooves staff development educators to determine if an offering should be presented on a centralized basis if the output (performance behavior) does not reflect attainment of the stated objectives. In other words, all factors should be considered before accepting centralization as economical, efficient, and effective.

Unfortunately, many people regard the number of offerings available or the number of people attending the offerings as the basis of a "good, economical effort." However, in any centralized effort, careful consideration must be given to the content that will facilitate employees' assuming their roles in the agency. Frequently the experience cannot be adequately gained solely through a centralized approach.

Several advantages accrue from a centralized approach. Administration can place responsibility and accountability more specifically with the staff development director and can scrutinize more closely the budget and the evaluation. If the number of staff development educators is limited, a better utilization of their efforts may result. A centralized approach also offers more uniformity in the implementation of standards.

A failure to meet the real needs may occur when input from the learners is not given adequate consideration in the planning or presentation of the learning offerings. It is possible to incorporate individualization in centralized programs, but it may not be so pronounced as in decentralized situations. Because learning needs do vary in different clinical areas, the centralized approach that offers broad-based, generalized content may not be adequate in all situations and may need to be supplemented by content that focuses on specific learning needs related to an employee's particular clinical area.

To assess whether a centralized staff development program is responsive to needs and remains viable under changing conditions, the following questions concerning the factors of economy, efficiency, and coordinated efforts must be asked:

- Does it provide staff development for *all* personnel?
- Does it respond rapidly and effectively to learning needs?
- Does it promote relevancy of learning to practice?
- Does it readily allow for the introduction of a new program?
- Does it provide a structure that delineates accountability for the various components?

If the answers are an unequivocable "yes," the current structure is probably suitable for meeting the needs of the employees. If not, the discrepancies need to be analyzed. Depending on the responses to these questions in relation to the particular situation, needs, and goals, it may be advisable to consider a decentralized or centralized-decentralized approach.

Decentralized approach

The concept of decentralization recognizes that the right to decide or the authority to make a decision is inherent in the performance of selected activities or tasks. Thus staff development educators are organized within clinical areas and are responsible for meeting the learning needs of a more circumscribed group of employees.

Timing and relevancy, essential factors in the teaching-learning process, can be applied more readily in a decentralized approach. Because the staff development educators are involved more directly in clinical situations, they generally can identify learning needs more rapidly. They also can pinpoint specific needs relevant to the clinical situation. We have found that some learners are unable to transfer general concepts into specific clinical situations. With decentralization the general concepts can be interpreted in specific ways for the given clinical situation.

The process of socialization is also enhanced in a decentralized approach. Identification with and acceptance by the learners' work group versus identification with a centralized representative or being a "face in the crowd" may affect the readiness to learn. In a decentralized approach, greater rewards will probably be achieved in terms of change in behavior (performance) through opportunities for individual goal setting, planning individually prescribed learning systems, capitalizing on the "teachable moments," and the presence of immediate reward or reinforcement systems. The involvement of more people in the process also frequently results in a greater commitment to the total effort and can lead to a "spread effect," because assisting others in development also helps individuals to develop themselves.

Centralized-decentralized approach

A combined centralized-decentralized approach utilizes certain aspects from each structure. It offers the option of having a degree of centralization necessary for planning and policy development in coordination with a decentralized clinical "learning operation." This approach recognizes the goals of the agency as a whole as well as the particular needs of its various parts.

Learning needs related to the participants' acquiring a common body of knowledge and skills may be met through a centralized learning offering, for instance, measuring temperature, pulse, and respirations. Concomitantly, those learning needs requiring an individual to acquire a range of specialized skills and to demonstrate these skills may be planned on a decentralized basis.

It is recognized that conditions conducive to producing effective outcomes include (1) having an opportunity to assume the new role initially under supervised practice, (2) having an opportunity to acquire proficiency in the skills, and (3) having feedback and guidance on performance as the "new" pattern of behavior is acquired.

Early in their employment, nurses want to be involved in "nursing practice." Therefore it behooves the staff development educator to recognize this desire as a motivating force for incorporation of planned clinical learning experiences along with classroom efforts in any learning activity.

Implications for approach by nursing

In order to provide meaningful learning experiences in the context of ever-changing practices, a staff development educator must consider intra-agency as well as extra-agency factors that affect the whole orientation of nursing practice. The following changes are affecting the dimensions of nursing and are relevant to the approach taken in meeting the learning needs of nurses and the nursing staff.

1. The changing role and functions of the professional nurse in the health care system
2. Changing patient care patterns
3. New technology
4. Nursing service organizations with:
   a. Decentralization of authority
   b. Relief from nonnursing duties
   c. Introduction of nurse clinicians
5. A move toward development of goals related to a specific nursing area and then to the broader agency goals (the "management by objectives" [MBO] concept)
6. Change in management practices as the needs of both workers and managers are clarified (participative management)
7. Research in nursing practice resulting in new and improved ways of providing nursing care

In view of the increasing demands for accountability, staff development educators must be cognizant of their responsibility as professional persons in providing learning offerings. The characteristics of today's nursing practice and the view that nursing education is a continuing process require that the nurse be given an opportunity to participate in relevant and timely learning activities. Although many agencies still provide only centralized learning offerings, the trend toward programming on a centralized-decentralized basis is growing. In a clinical area the head nurse, supervisor, or nurse clinician can be the role model, create a climate for learning, and implement an individualized plan based on the learners' levels of proficiency in relation to the current demands of their particular roles. These expectations of behaviors required in a clinical situation are fulfilled more readily in the specific setting. A clinical-based experience can facilitate learning because it allows for understanding of the consequences and encourages continuing efforts and successful innovations. Because the learners see the results of their actions within their respective clinical areas, there are greater opportunities for reinforcement of positive behavior. The completion of the basic nursing program provides only the initial and minimum requirements for practice, making it necessary that each nurse participate in continuing education to keep skills and competencies up to date.[3] Although what the agency offers is crucial, it is no longer totally adequate. For the various reasons cited, it is important to consider use of all available learning resources to improve the quality of care.

APPROACHES TO ORGANIZING STAFF DEVELOPMENT

There are a number of ways in which the staff development function may be organized. In a large, complex agency the responsibility for staff development for nursing may be a function at the nursing administrative level. If the agency and the departments are decentralized, the authority and accountability for staff development may be assigned to an educator in the clinical area who usually has equal status to other administrative personnel in the area (Fig. 5-1). The title for such a position might be director of staff development, assistant director for staff development, or coordinator of staff development. In this organizational approach the staff development administrator would report directly to the nursing administrator and have responsibility for broad functions such as planning, implementing, and evaluating the centralized components of orientation and continuing education; providing consultation services on a decentralized basis for identification of learning needs; initiating offerings to meet learning

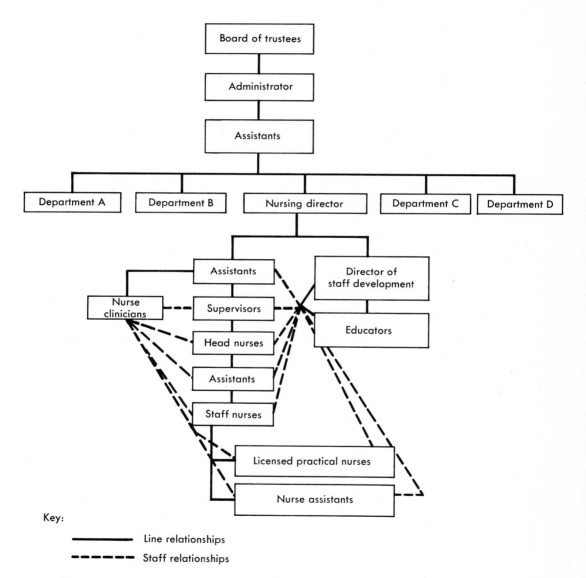

Key:

—————— Line relationships

▬ ▬ ▬ ▬ ▬ Staff relationships

Fig. 5-1. Agency organizational chart with staff development within the nursing department. In a large, complex agency the responsibility for staff development for nursing may be assigned to an administrative nursing position that is usually of equal status with assistant directors.

needs; providing resource and reference materials; and assisting colleagues in other ways in the implementation of decentralized learning offerings. An instructional staff may be assigned solely on a centralized basis or on a centralized and decentralized basis.

A trend in some agencies is to assign the function of staff development to an agency-wide education department (Fig. 5-2). This approach has primarily gained momentum from the recognition that continuing education is needed by all personnel if they are to keep pace with rapid change. Nursing staff development is one of the major components of this organizational approach. Essential in this plan is the clear understanding that nursing personnel are responsible for the identification of their individual learning needs.

A third method of organizing staff development is also within the clinical area (Fig.

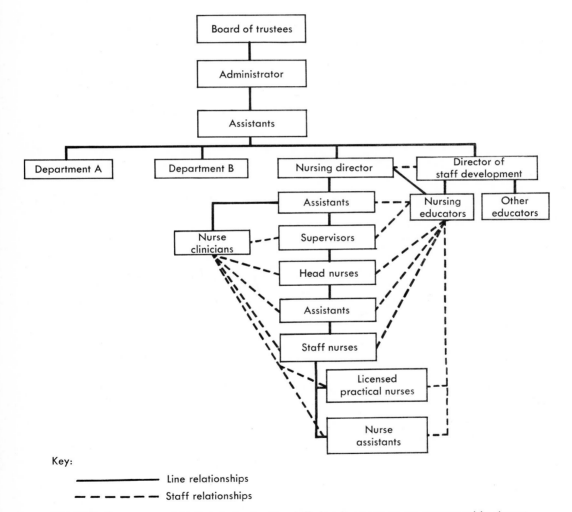

Key:

——————————— Line relationships

— — — — — — Staff relationships

Fig. 5-2. Agency organizational chart with staff development as an agency-wide department. Within this framework the department of staff development has a formal relationship with the nursing department. The nursing practice aspect of staff development originates from the nursing department, not from the staff development department.

5-3). In this approach, each educator is assigned a specific clinical area and is accountable to the clinical leader. The staff development educators hold staff positions in the clinical setting and are responsible for learning opportunities in their defined areas. All of the educators are linked to the director of staff development in terms of overall planning and coordination.

ORGANIZATION PATTERNS OF COMMITTEES

One approach to the organization of staff development that has proved effective in many agencies involves the use of committees. Where there are a limited number of staff development educators, this approach might be considered as one source of additional support. However, committees may be useful in any size agency with any number of

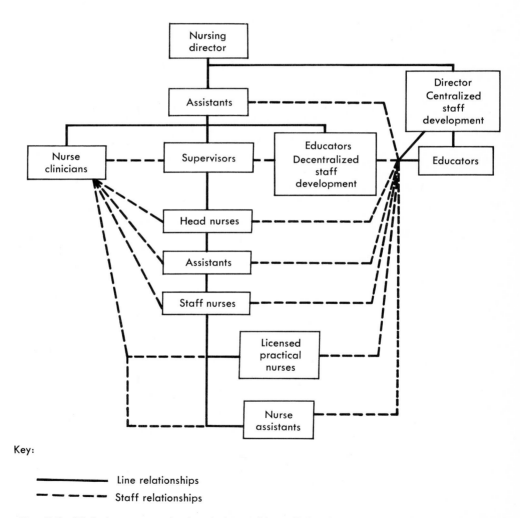

Key:

——————— Line relationships

— — — — — Staff relationships

Fig. 5-3. Clinical area organizational chart with staff development on a centralized-decentralized basis. There is a relationship for overall planning and coordination with the director of centralized staff development while facilitating attainment of goals within the clinical area.

instructors. A committee is organized and operates to achieve a purpose; therefore it has a decision-making or advisory capacity. The real point of differentiation between the two is in the authority and function of the group, the former having authority to make decisions and act and the latter providing counseling or making recommendations.

If a committee approach is elected, it is wise to develop the guidelines in advance. These include defining the committee's goal or purpose, functions, authority, the individual to whom it reports and is accountable, and the membership (with regard to requirements of eligibility, selection, term of appointment, and replacement of members). The purpose of the committee should influence the number and type of individuals appointed to it. For instance, if a standing committee were appointed to plan and present a specific learning offering, it probably would require appointment of members having specific competencies, backgrounds, or interests.

A committee may be either temporary or standing. An ad hoc or temporary committee is appointed for a specific purpose and is disbanded once that purpose is achieved. It usually arises from a new or current necessity that has not or cannot be dealt with within the existing structure. For example, an ad hoc committee might be created to study the charting system; when the group makes a recommendation or reaches the decision it becomes defunct. If, however, one of the purposes is implementation of changes, the committee would remain in existence until this purpose was accomplished as well. This type of committee is usually concerned with a single problem or situation. However, it may require a more concerted effort on the part of its members because of its temporary status.

A standing committee has a permanent place in the organization and thus is identified in organization charts. It has more permanent functions and usually deals with continuing, broader-based problems or activities. Because of its broad functions, it continues until it is no longer appropriate. For example, a committee may be established to review and revise all nursing procedures. Because this is a never-ending task, the committee would most likely be a standing one. It is doubtful that it would become extinct unless the decision was made to establish a different mechanism for the task. It may be necessary to have both an advisory and planning committee to deal with both aspects on a continuing basis.

Advisory committee

The membership of an advisory committee may or may not represent a broad background of knowledge, attitudes, and experiences. For example, nurses from various clinical areas and types of nursing (registered nurses as well as licensed practical nurses), the nursing administrators, and the director of staff development would constitute a well-rounded advisory group. The committee's functions would be to (1) provide overall advice and guidance in planning activities, (2) review and evaluate the ongoing program and operating functions, (3) promote coordination, collaboration, and communication among the nursing groups, (4) promote implementation of recommendations, (5) consider any proposed program or learning offerings in terms of need and program design, and (6) assist in establishing priorities. The advisory committee should also look to the future. It may want to plan experimental programs for application at a later date. In order to plan for future needs of the agency, the advisory committee might recommend health manpower studies to determine if a restructuring of jobs would improve utilization of the available manpower.

This committee could also recommend policies governing staff development. Such decisions might pertain to whether attendance is mandatory or voluntary, the frequency of certain programs, the responsibility for promoting the offerings, required records and reports, the process of evaluation, and compensation for those attending staff development offerings.

Planning committee

The planning committee should have a broader range than the advisory committee in both membership and function. The membership ought to include representatives from the various clinical areas, the administrators for the nursing care programs, and representatives from the various shifts who are involved in implementing changes. This latter category includes not only line personnel but also those staff members who serve as role models and initiators of action in specific clinical areas. In essence, the group must represent the real world of practice—individuals who can articulate why an approach will not work, what changes need to be made to facilitate a new approach, and how specific groups will be affected by the planned changes. These individuals must also have a commitment to change and the means with which to achieve it. Thus when a staff member is alert to the various factors involved in change but cannot effect it because of poor relations with the nursing staff, another individual who can compensate for this implementation deficiency should perhaps be added. However, the committee must not become so big that its effectiveness is diminished by the number of people involved. On the other hand, if there are not enough people involved, the recommendations may be relevant to only one area rather than to the entire agency. If a large number of people are to be included, a basic planning committee might be established, with the others serving as resource people to the committee members. The planning committee has responsibility for overall design and makes the final decision on a program or learning offering. Although the functions may include approving policies, delegating authority for the program, seeking ways to support activities, and participating in the evaluation process, they will be dependent on the organization of the committee and the leadership styles of its members.

Staff development educator's responsibility

The staff development educator should preside over the planning committee and serve as a member or the chairman of the advisory committee. The role of chairman would encompass planning and preparing the agenda, providing any necessary advance data needed, applying group dynamics, and communicating in writing to the appropriate authority (probably the director of nursing) with regard to the committee's activities, concerns, actions, and recommendations.

A variety of techniques may be employed to promote committee attendance and participation: (1) meeting dates are set and notices sent out in advance, (2) an agenda of the meeting is determined in advance and stated on the meeting notice, (3) advance information is sent with the notice and agenda, (4) minutes are recorded, and (5) a protocol is determined for recording and reporting the committee's recommendations.

If attendance is inconsistent or sporadic, it becomes very difficult for the committee to reach its full potential. Also, if one member is constantly absent, this input is lost.

Minutes are taken during the meeting by an appointed recorder. The final minutes are usually prepared following the meeting. The minutes should include the following items: (1) information such as name of the committee, date, time, place, when the meeting was called to order, members present (including titles if appropriate), and the name of the presiding officer and (2) the body of the minutes—a brief chronological record of agenda items, rationale for decisions if appropriate, a record of discussions, and actions taken or business transacted. Use of general headings and subheadings in the margin to the left of the related content can prove helpful. Minutes are usually signed by the recorder and sent to members as soon as they are prepared. They are corrected or approved at the following meeting.

FORMULATION OF POLICIES AND PROCEDURES

The formulation of policies and procedures involves an agreement on what is expected. Each policy is a guideline for the decisions or actions of the people in the agency. The aim of a policy is to effectively influence the performance of the individuals. In addition to identifying the accountability of individuals, policies also establish certain parameters within a given setting. For example, staff development policies define the manner in which learning is to be offered, to whom it applies, under what conditions it is relevant, and the specific focus of the issue. Policies are usually in writing but may be unwritten (implied) if they have arisen as a result of practice over a period of time. When a policy is not stated in writing, but its existence is evident in observable behaviors of employees, it is known as an implied policy. While implied policies may be of benefit, they may also create problems.

Procedures explain the "how to" of the policy. They are usually developed in a sequential manner to indicate the agency's accepted approach to a particular task. For example, within staff development the policy regarding mandatory attendance at safety programs might have a related procedure outlining the maintenance of records and reports.

Policies as well as procedures guide the staff development educator in attaining staff development goals. Policies having maximum scope are administered from the top, and those with a more narrow and specific application are administered at a lower level; an overall policy might make all safety programs mandatory for all nursing personnel, while a particular unit may require that its employees attend the CPR drills every six months.

Policies at the operational level (clinical areas) must be consistent with and supportive of the higher level policies if the structure is to be effective. When this interrelation of policy does not exist, problems may arise in implementation. The aim of policies is to obtain uniformity of action. In implementing policies, consideration must be given to such related factors as flexibility, consistency, fairness, and judgment. The degrees of centralization and decentralization in the agency determine how the policies are formulated and initiated.

Policies may be arrived at by consensus or by administrative decision. The agency nurs-ing administration may adopt broad and general policies for employees. An example of a broad policy would be that all employees must attend the agency's orientation program. However, this is not to say that this same policy might not come by consensus. If, for example, head nurses agreed that all nursing personnel were not performing emergency resuscitation measures correctly, they may decide by consensus that reorientation is necessary. Greater support can be gained if the nursing administration agrees with this decision. Within the framework of the broad departmental policies, staff development may define those policies needed to accomplish the learning functions, while the head nurses may establish the policy for the unit staff. For example, the staff development educators may determine a prerequisite for the learners such as previous attendance at a leadership workshop. The head nurses may establish the policy that seniority and availability of the individual determine who among those qualified may attend.

The process of developing policies consists of a joint effort between staff development educators and the clinical staff. A policy might be based on the mitigating factors that influence its enforcement. For instance, the hour(s) of offerings could be defined but, if the staffing pattern and the staff work load would not permit attendance, the effectiveness of the policy would be diminished. Without clinical support the performance behaviors may not be readily identified.

Additionally, other groups may need to become involved in the development of policy statements as the physician-nurse roles and relationships change. Some of these changing functions are involved with the development of interdependent roles. Thus the resultant policy should be enforced equally by both groups. The predicted extension and expansion of nursing roles would indicate that this type of policy statement will be seen more frequently.

Initially, policies need to be defined and established to show how the desired goals of staff development are to be achieved. Because a policy forms the basis on which decisions are made, the initial policies probably will be formulated for purposes of defining attendance and participation in the learning offerings. Additional policies may need to be written at a later date when discrepancies or recurring problems become evident.

Although determination of the overall policies is an administrative responsibility, the need for a policy may arise at the operational level. In a decentralized organization the operational level probably will have more influence on policy development than it would in a centralized setting. Therefore staff nurses could expect more input in the former situation than in the latter.

The effectiveness of policy implementation is affected directly by the existing communication channels. Because they must be interpreted and implemented by the line personnel, policies should be in writing and available to all employees. Policies may be disseminated in a number of ways. They may be issued in the form of written statements, bulletins, manuals, handbooks, or as news releases. Use of such materials as colored paper, pages with a colored border, or a specific design may serve as a cue for employees. For example, a communication with a colored border may indicate that attendance is required.

While verbal announcements or responses may be made, this method involves the highest risk of misinterpretation. Written policies offer the following advantages: (1) they are available to all in the same form, (2) they can be utilized as a reference, and (3) they can be made available to all who are affected by them. For example, giving new employees copies of staff development policies that are applicable to them may provide an incentive for them to participate in certain learning offerings.

Policies in staff development are written for a specific purpose and the content reflects that purpose. For example, the policies formulated will relate primarily to attendance and participation: whether it is voluntary or required, on a privileged or selected basis, compensated or not, and open or closed. (See Appendix, Exhibit A.)

FACILITIES AND RESOURCES

In order to conduct learning offerings within an agency, the physical facilities, the physical resources, the financial resources, and the human resources must be considered. Each is significant in its own right as well as affecting the other three factors. The staff development philosophy and goals provide a basis for planning and determine the facilities and resources to be secured. The planning process incorporates relationships that presently exist among and within areas that have learning offerings or provide educational services in the agency. Criteria for facilities and resources should be defined in advance and used as plans are developed. An example of some typical standards appears in Table 5-1.

Facilities

Planning objectives may be based on operational objectives such as the following:
1. Acquire facilities designed to permit the application of adult learning concepts.
2. Acquire adequate teaching, office, and storage space to meet the needs.
3. Develop a flexible physical structure to promote versatility.

These objectives would have several effects. First, they recognize the importance of establishing an environment conducive to adult learning. Physical aspects such as ventilation, seating arrangements, and a pleasant setting are cited as important to adults when they are in "learner" roles. Additionally, the teaching areas should accommodate individuals as well as small and large groups. These areas may include classrooms, lecture-demonstration areas, conference and seminar rooms, multipurpose rooms, and study areas. The scheduling and utilization of the facility should be considered in determining needs. The roles of the staff development educators determine the placement of their offices; for

Table 5-1. Standards for facilities and resources

Standard	Rationale
Facilities are sufficient in numbers and type to provide the essential learning experiences for the learners.	The size and availability of a facility can influence the method of teaching. Various settings are needed for individual and group learning.
The physical facilities and the organizational structure are conducive to effective use.	Physical aspects such as ventilation, seating arrangements, size, and sound have an influence on the learning situation.
Teaching technology is available as needed.	Adequate hardware and software, which are accessible and appropriate to the learning need, supplement the educator's use of self.
Secretarial assistance of sufficient quantity and quality is available.	The secretarial staff assists in the preparation of agency materials and in the maintenance of necessary records and reports.
There is a system for storage, maintenance, and use of equipment and for the control of supplies and reference materials.	Maintaining a control system facilitates reduced maintenance.
The budget is sufficient to support the staff development goals.	Adequate financing includes not only present needs but also projections for future goals.
The staff development educators are available to all learners.	The objectives of the various offerings influence the number of staff development educators and their assignment.

instance, in a decentralized setting an office may be adjacent to the clinical area. Storage space that allows for accessibility and proper controls should be established. A library facility that is accessible and has current reference materials is necessary. If special projects are assumed by the staff, a "work room" needs to be considered.

Facilities should be flexible enough to meet a variety of needs. New devices and changes can be incorporated more readily if the basic facilities are adaptable. The kinds of offerings to be presented, the types of learning experiences to be provided, and the frequency of such offerings provide the operational framework for determining the adequacy or inadequacy of the facility. Initial questions in determining needs may be "Will offerings be formal or informal?" "What basic learning offerings will be provided on a regular basis?"

"What teaching methods will be used?"

Depending on the content, the methods, and the learners, the facilities should accommodate different kinds of learning activities such as lectures, demonstrations, and return demonstrations. If the orientation involves an average of ten nurses and the teaching methods include lectures, demonstrations, use of audiovisual aids, and individual learning systems, then a facility that permits different seating arrangements, visibility when different visual media are used, and some privacy would be advisable. If a demonstration and return demonstration of a patient care technique were planned, then a laboratory setting might be deemed more desirable. Two ways to achieve flexibility are to have large, free spaces or portable partitions that readily allow for change in the facility. Portable rather than fixed equipment may be used in various ways also. Projected plans may also include the use of computer terminals and closed-circuit television.

In recent years the shift from a centralized to a decentralized program has tended to redirect the focus of teaching efforts. In addition, with the change in staffing patterns in nursing areas, establishing learning offerings that can be utilized near the clinical area becomes necessary. Conference rooms located in or adjacent to clinical areas provide space for the pursuit of decentralized staff development. Installation of learning carrels for computer-assisted instruction in nursing areas also offers learning opportunities for individualized pursuit.

In developing a facility, it is advisable to prepare a number of different designs at the outset. As indicated earlier, the planning process should involve several individuals, including the staff development educators. The different designs will indicate the overall physical structure, desired features, and furnishings of the facility.

A checklist of factors that are pertinent to the needs may give some direction in planning. The following factors are interrelated:

1. Size. How large a group will it accommodate?
2. Lighting. Is it adequate for the particular learning activities?
3. Visibility. Will everyone be able to see what is going on?
4. Acoustics. Are outside noises a possible distracting factor?
5. Electrical outlets. Are they of the right type, properly located, and adequate for the operation of audiovisual equipment?
6. Windows and window coverings. Do they permit light as well as allow for room darkening?
7. Storage space. Does it offer sufficient space for equipment and materials? Can security be effected if necessary?
8. Furnishings. Which type (movable, fixed, or a combination) is needed? Is a work surface area (arm-type seating

tables, carrels) required? Is a display system needed?

After reviewing the various possibilities, a design should be selected for recommendation. Follow-up plans for later expansion may also be defined at the present time. The next step in completing the design is deciding on the dimensions of the movable equipment and determining if it can be utilized within the given space. The design should take into account efficiency and labor-saving factors. It should incorporate a method for accommodation to physical change. Mechanical devices such as temperature and humidity controls should be included.

Physical resources

Teaching devices that can be purchased or rented and that should be considered basic include a movie projector, slide projector, film strip projector, screen, overhead projector, display board, photostat or duplicating equipment, and tape recorder. In order to determine what is needed in terms of additional equipment, the individual situation must be analyzed. Just because some other agency bought a particular piece of equipment or because there is one excellent item of software with some particular system provides no justification for purchase.

Keeping records of the utilization of facilities and equipment will be helpful in projecting future needs. For example, maintaining sign-up sheets for the use of equipment or classrooms provides data on use and the need for more space or additional equipment. Without this information there may be difficulty in obtaining additional space and equipment.

Establishing a system for the selection of equipment and supplies is linked to the budgetary process because of the expenditures involved. Having a data base of usage patterns and the scope of the maintenance services can assist in the selection of new equipment. A program of preventive maintenance and an orientation process to the operation and control of the equipment should also be established. Chapter 9 deals with the types of hardware and software most likely to be used in staff development. The choice of such equipment will depend on the needs and budget.

Financial resources

The budget may be described as a plan of financial operations that has been agreed on and approved for a definite period of time. Budgets are tools in financial planning, coordinating, and control, the purposes of which are (1) to provide a review of financial requirements; (2) to reflect demands for an increase or an expansion in costs for the learning offerings, personnel, equipment, and supplies that may have been identified during or since the initial planning phases of staff development; (3) to provide a financial mechanism for the establishment of new offerings; and (4) to provide a comparison of actual with projected costs of the personnel, equipment, and services.

Some type of accounting system is a prerequisite to budgeting. In many agencies the various departments are involved in the budgeting process. For example, the director of nursing may coordinate all the budgetary plans of the nursing divisions into a financial program for the department.

Staff development educators should have an understanding of their responsibilities in planning, evaluating, and controlling the fiscal activities of staff development. Their role expectations include defining the needs for equipment, supplies, services, and personnel for the coming year. In planning the budget there is some degree of involvement by the educational staff. They participate in the planning that is related to their specific responsibilities. For example, the educators who have responsibility for the orientation program would provide input about equipment, supplies, and services needed for that program during the next fiscal year. The budgetary process also may offer the opportunity for long-term planning; some agencies incorporate long-term planning and goal setting

as well as the projection of immediate budgetary needs.

Usually budgetary requests are submitted on forms provided by the administration, who also sets a timetable for the preparation and submission of the preliminary budget. The overall budgetary process includes discussion, review, and decision making leading to a final determination.

Factors that may influence the need to add equipment or increase the personnel include an expanded nursing care program that requires learning offerings because of new or changing roles or a shift in functions from one area to another that increases the skills needed by the personnel assigned to the area.

There are four basic areas to be included in a budget—personnel, capital expenditures, equipment, and supplies. Depending on the approach used by the agency, it will be necessary to delineate the number and types of personnel needed and their salaries. In some agencies it is also necessary to compute the fringe benefits such as sick leave, vacation, and insurance. In other agencies this information is calculated on the basis of the salary and classification of employees. Generally the amount of money to be allocated for educational and professional expenses should be indicated. Documentation of the need for additional staff should be given in support of the request.

The capital expenditures budget also varies among agencies. In some agencies, items costing over a hundred dollars may be included in this part of the nursing department budget; however, in other agencies the sum may be more. Some agencies view anything "fixed to the wall" as a part of this budget. Hence renovation expenses would be included here. Most items in this budget have long-range implications and therefore need to be justified in the budget sessions. It is helpful to have data to support the outlay of large amounts of money.

Equipment includes the hardware essential to the program of staff development. Because the selection of a piece of hardware can "lock" the agency into that particular system, caution must be exercised in the selection of items. Basically an item should be durable, portable, easily repairable, adaptable, and usable. If the first four aspects are present, but the item is very difficult to use, it may become a "white elephant." The costs for these items should be projected in the budget in terms of a new or replacement item. Again, justification may be necessary.

In many agencies, furnishings are included in this budget. Furniture for offices and classrooms are typical examples. Depending on how the budget is determined in a specific agency, the educational furnishings on nursing units may also be included. For example, two nursing units may need to install learning carrels for the personnel and patients and these items might be incorporated in this budget.

In both the capital expenditures and equipment budgets there are usually costs related to depreciation of the items and to maintenance expenses. Generally it is not the responsibility of the staff development educators to determine these costs. However, these factors should be taken into account.

Finally, the supplies budget includes software, references, and the usual office necessities. Software requirements are based on the available hardware. In some agencies, references may be a part of a library budget, while in others they are included in the staff development budget. Generally the references on the various nursing units are assigned to the respective budgets. The typical office supplies (paper, pencils, stencils or mimeograph, carbon paper, binders, folders, etc.) should be projected in terms of what was used in a preceding period and what the needs are likely to be in the future. Many agencies produce a computerized printout of costs to date on a regular basis that provides a fairly accurate picture of current expenditures.

Planned program budgeting. The planned program budgeting system is an approach being taken in many agencies and is considered a more responsive and effective system for decision makers. Better decisions can be made on the basis of facts and data. Basically, planned program budgeting involves the establishment of objectives in quantifiable terms, consideration of all costs and benefits, and analysis of the objectives and alternatives over an adequate time period. An example might be the development of more extensive teaching technology to meet certain needs. All items must be determined in terms of costs and benefits to the consumers, for instance, that the outlay of so many dollars for a particular piece of equipment will allow patients and personnel on individual nursing units to learn up-to-date information about certain health conditions. It is necessary to set a time limit for accomplishing the objective.

Human resources

One of the most valuable assets an agency has is its human resources. As previously mentioned, the budget must support the maintenance of the necessary staff.

Staffing is a process by which individuals are assigned to positions. It might be considered as having as its central purpose the achievement of staff development goals. The ultimate responsibility for staff development lies with the director or nursing, but the delegation of functions depends on the situation and the human resources available. The functions of staff development may be assigned to an individual, to administrative personnel assigned to clinical areas, or to a committee. However, the administrative functions must be assigned specifically and the responsibility and authority for staff development must be delineated and defined in the written position description. One of the major factors to consider is the organizational structure of the department. The following questions must be considered:

- What is the process of planning and decision making in the nursing department?
- Is the organizational structure highly centralized or decentralized, or do both patterns exist?
- Does decision making come only from the

director of nursing, or do the head nurses have authority and responsibility for establishing priorities and making decisions relative to nursing practice?

• Where is the administrative control up and down the line of the structure, and what are the organizational relationships?

The administrative responsibility includes determining the number and qualifications of the staff development educators.

Determining staffing requirements. To place staffing in proper perspective one must know the functions of staff development, the manpower data base of the agency, the role changes emerging now and those anticipated in the future, and the impact of technology. The functions of staff development may include the following:

1. Establishing a system that provides for the input of the staff development process
2. Identifying learning needs utilizing a number of ways and collaborative processes
3. Providing and evaluating learning offerings to meet these needs
4. Maintaining a communications system that incorporates the use of media in such a way as to encourage and foster participation, involvement, and cooperation
5. Formulating an organizational structure to make the system operate in such a way that facilities and resources are utilized to accomplish the overall and specific objectives of the learning offerings and to meet changing needs
6. Participating in the development and updating of the philosophy, objectives, policies, procedures, position descriptions, and performance appraisal systems for nursing service
7. Making appropriate applications of research and study findings to staff development programming
8. Conducting studies and research activities related to the utilization and development of human resources
9. Disseminating information about relevant learning offerings within and outside the agency to the nursing staff
10. Maintaining a system of records and reports for staff development
11. Coordinating the utilization of nursing areas by educational and other institutions
12. Developing and utilizing an evaluation process that is ongoing and is applied to all elements of the staff development process
13. Promoting a positive learning climate
14. Selecting or developing media (hardware and software) that are appropriate and feasible for learning offerings
15. Developing and implementing a budget

The concepts of timing, relevancy, and continuity also influence staffing requirements. The concept of timing requires that the offering be in line with what the employees are currently doing or will do in the near future. For example, if there is evidence that an increased number of patients with cardiac monitors will be assigned throughout the medical service, the need to prepare the staff nurses to provide care in these circumstances can be met before the fact. Relevancy is concerned with relating the content to the employee's learning needs and role expectations as opposed to content of a general or unrelated nature. Continuity implies that the staff is available to plan and implement the offerings on a continuing basis to reinforce positive learning. In other words, without adequate resources and planning time there can be failure in one or all of these aspects.

Use of a manpower data base is one approach that may be taken in planning for staffing. Past appointments and attrition rates are reviewed and the approach is one of demand and supply.[4] The scheduling of orientation programs that have quality control and cost effectiveness may be a problem when this approach is used; the availability of nurses is an intervening variable in the demand-supply approach. Some alternatives in orientation program scheduling might be to conduct programs on a regular basis regardless of the number of appointments; appoint nurses when they are available for vacant positions and provide primarily an individualized orientation; or provide all orientation on a decentralization basis. The pros and cons of each alternative would need to be weighed, the approach always being consistent with the goals.

Staffing options. Whether staffing is a problem in the agency or not, some teaching options should be considered. The extent of the needs, goals, and parameters of the policies will assist in determining how they are to be employed.

Option 1: Opportunity for utilization of individually prescribed learning systems. This approach should be given high priority, as it allows individuals to pace themselves in learning and provides recognition of their abilities.

Option 2: Provision of a core program with career tracks. This approach permits individuals to pursue career patterns within the agency according to their interest and capabilities. A core program in which all agency employees participate could assist in their recognizing the contributions each of them makes to the delivery of patient care. For example, a case presentation may serve several purposes in providing discussion for physicians, nurses, pharmacists, and physical therapists.

Option 3: Provision of pretests in selected learning offerings. Pretests provide the staff development educator with an indication of what is needed by the learners. They also alert the learners to areas of discrepancy.

Option 4: Provision of learning offerings that are sequential and build on each other. This approach allows for beginning and advanced programming to be planned in relation to learning needs. It can reduce learning time for those who possess advanced knowledge and skills. It also should be recognized

as eliminating the frustration or boredom that can occur when the content is already known.

Option 5: Provision of learning offerings having limited enrollment or specific criteria for enrollment. This might be at variance with overall needs but may produce highly desirable effects with a specific group.

Option 6: Provision of learning offerings that prepare individuals to assume responsibility for teaching others. This approach distributes the teaching responsibility. For example, certain aspects of diabetic teaching are amenable to this approach with nurse assistants.

Option 7: Offering opportunities to attend programs outside the agency. This may be practiced in promoting the maintenance of a viable agency or in meeting specific kinds of learning needs.

Option 8: Bringing in resources or sharing services and resources. These approaches may supplement or complement programming. Success in this approach usually relates to having common interests and goals.

Option 9: Utilization of allied health professionals. Professionals from other disciplines may function as assistants to the educator in selected activities. These persons can be utilized in such a way that everyone benefits.

Another factor in planning for staff development is related to the rapid changes in roles and role relationships in the health care team. The staff development educator must be flexible in order to respond to new demands.

Selection of staff. Selection of staff involves finding those individuals most capable of directing their efforts toward the attainment of the agency's goals. The selection process consists of the same techniques that are applied to any professional applicant. If applicants are presently functioning in other roles, the process may be broadened to include observation of specific performances such as the ability to apply teaching-learning principles in staff- and patient-education situations. The process of selecting the right person is a complex one. Essential qualities may differ with regard to agency size, available resources, and what the role will be.

Criteria for appointment to the position should be established through a delineation of the abilities, skills, and experience required. Certain aspects may be emphasized in the selection process. Two important criteria are knowledge and skill in the clinical area as well as adult learning. In order to serve as effective teachers, it is desirable for staff development educators to be expert in some particular area in addition to being generalists in the field of nursing. Because the learners are adults, it is equally important for the educational staff to be aware of adult learning concepts.

Depending on the setting, the staff development educators may be prepared at various educational levels. Generally someone with considerably fewer qualifications than the learners should not be expected to bring about change unless that individual is particularly skillful. Registered nurses normally comprise the staff, although other personnel may be used for specific types of offerings.

Personal characteristics that are desirable include a desire to learn, as exemplified by the individual's pursuit of learning opportunities; a zeal for helping others to learn; a willingness to accept responsibility; and the qualities of being receptive to change, new ideas, and experimentation. Having the ability to work with others on a basis of mutual respect, understanding, and cooperation is important because staff development educators should attempt to influence employees without coercion. Staff development educators must believe in the importance of staff development for the agency, be aware of the problems and needs of nursing services, and be creative and imaginative. Further, they need to be able to accept rewards indirectly; their effectiveness is reflected by the demonstrated behavior changes in head nurses and others in such a way that the change itself seems to be their own idea rather than that of the staff development educator. Based on the premise that human resources are the most valuable asset of an agency, it follows that selection of the right individuals can assist in offsetting other deficiencies that might exist in the program.

Other types of staff may include secretaries and audiovisual experts. The secretaries must be able to produce quality work, usually in a large volume. They need to be skilled in typing, filing, record-keeping, and taking some form of dictation to increase the educators' efficiency in communication.

Many agencies have begun to use audiovisual experts to assist in developing and maintaining hardware and software. If these teaching aids are relied on, it might be advantageous to have an expert on the scene. While it is important to know the usual techniques in preparing and repairing standard hardware and software, it is not a major responsibility and can be time-consuming. Additionally, an audiovisual technician can help to create those aids that will be most useful in a particular learning offering.

ROLES AND RELATIONSHIPS OF STAFF DEVELOPMENT EDUCATORS

Staff development educators usually occupy staff positions. The personnel of an agency may be divided into the categories of line and staff. The line personnel have the authority and the responsibility to achieve results. A line position allows actions to be produced on the issuance of an order or by supervision of activities. On the other hand, a staff position is advisory in nature and provides a service to the line personnel, therefore facilitating the work of the line. Responsibilities in staff development efforts should be defined as clearly as possible, although some responsibilities will necessarily be shared. A communications network is essential, and staff development educators may deem it necessary to keep informed through formal channels of communication. Individual conferences with the director of nursing could be scheduled on a regular basis if needed.

The staff development director implements a planning process that consistently identifies and evaluates strategic options. Performance requirements include responsibility for the administrative functions of planning, organizing, directing, influencing, and supporting the work of others and applying nursing, adult learning, and change theories in the organization and administration of the staff development efforts. Direction must also be given to learning-management systems so that optimization of resources, learning activities, and individual performance behavior occurs.

Role expectations for the staff development educator include the following:

1. Identifying learning needs for particular learning offerings as well as general learning offerings
2. Planning for the learning offerings that will lead to the desired behavior
3. Defining approaches and alternatives to meet needs
4. Setting a climate
5. Determining the media and teaching strategies for assisting the individuals to attain the desired behaviors
6. Securing the resources (human and other) that are needed
7. Evaluating the process on an ongoing basis

The role is that of a *facilitator or resource* rather than a "giver of information." Planning learning activities that require experience or supervised practice in the clinical area involves joint planning and sharing of information with the clinical personnel. In addition, regular meetings with the head nurse should be set up so that any problems can be identified and discussed and new learning situations can be determined. Written information pertinent to scheduling and to the "learners" should be provided to the nursing area.

Assignment of staff

The staff may be assigned in one of several ways—by components, shifts, classification of personnel, clinical expertise, teams, or differentiated staffing. Each approach incorporates specific responsibilities for the staff. There is no right or wrong way; it depends on the situation and the qualifications of the available persons.

As described in Chapter 8, staff development usually is divided into components to accomplish goals. Using our distinctions of orientation and continuing education, the staff would be assigned to one of these major efforts. This approach allows for development of knowledge and skills in a more circumscribed area. There is a potential hazard, however, if the educators do not assist with the other component. For example, in the clinical area there may be two educators—one for orientation and one for continuing education. This is confusing for the staff and should be avoided if possible.

A second approach in assigning staff is to have them designated by shifts (days, evenings, and nights). Although this approach allows the personnel on a shift to identify with an individual in terms of their learning needs, the educators may develop "tunnel" vision, seeing only a need or problem unique to their shifts. In addition, while this approach assures "'round-the-clock" coverage, it may not use the talents of the staff to their fullest potential.

Assignment by classification of personnel has been used in some agencies. In this approach the staff is divided among the categories of personnel in the department. Although the employees may benefit by associating with one specific individual who understands their role, the staff may be duplicating efforts in certain learning offerings. Also, they may develop separatist attitudes and not be able to recognize the importance of learning needs of other groups.

Clinical expertise as a basis for assignment allows for the use of the staffs' talents in the clinical area. Each educator is responsible for some major area, for example, maternal, medical-surgical, or cardiovascular nursing. Thus there would be a core of experts. It may be difficult to find individuals with the various clinical interests necessary to meet all the needs. The problem of separatism is possible with this approach also.

Team teaching is a concept that is applicable to staff development. This may be defined as a cooperative teaching effort between two or more educators where planning, presenting, and evaluating activities in a learning offering are shared on an ongoing basis with the premise that each educator has a purposeful intent. This approach provides the opportunity for built-in quality control. Team teaching also can be an interdisciplinary approach in which the resources and knowledge of health personnel are integrated. This integration can be a productive and meaningful approach in teaching certain content. For example, in a respiratory care program that includes content on drugs, the pharmacist could be utilized as a resource. Educators adopting the team approach may have less personal relationships with the learners and perhaps some difficulty in coordinating the total endeavor.

Differentiated staffing is another concept utilized in the field of education. The concept is based on the premise that within a given teacher population there are varying degrees of abilities and skills. These differences should be recognized in the development of innovations and in the decision making that affects the educational system. Therefore it is an approach that provides for a vertical career ladder. If this concept were applied within staff development, the educational staff would be organized so that different degrees of competency would be recognized. Boutwell[5] describes the process as defining the functions in terms of behaviors and placing them in a vertical career ladder. This concept places the staff in roles that would be differentiated in terms of teaching skills, knowledge, and leadership capabilities. As staff development educators increased their skills, they would advance within the staff development system. Implementation of this concept requires an evaluation process that includes peer as well as vertical review. Determining the number of appointments to each step of such a career ladder would require relating it to the learning needs within the agency so that over- or understaffing would not occur. As our need for sophisticated and innovative learning systems increases, the processes of planning and implementation require "talented" staff development educators who can effect relevant outcomes.

RECORDS AND REPORTS

The system of records and reports for staff development will differ according to the size and complexity of the agency and the functions of staff development. Further, the scope of the system will be affected by the requests for information from the nursing and agency administration, particular data needs within the agency, and the way in which information is used.

Records and reports are designed to provide the data base for the agency's information needs. Such documents serve a specific purpose in providing information concerning statistical data, documentation of activities, follow-up evaluation, and reference needs. Their value, however, lies in the kind and completeness of the information recorded. If staff development educators have a need for specific data, they may design a form for that purpose and identify the required data base. Before incorporating any specially designed record, the efforts needed to complete it and the economics involved in its use should be reviewed.

The records and reports commonly used in staff development are the master plan, the specific plans of the learning offerings, the annual report, interim report, individual employee and group records of attendance and achievement, statistical records, evaluations, budget records, and national or statewide standards.

Master plan

Formulating the master plan requires that the staff development educator look into the future and plan for it. For example, a master plan may assist in unifying and coordinating plans and in scheduling specific learning offerings that arise from a major policy, for instance, new nursing employees may start every two weeks. This plan serves as a framework for specific programming, allows for assignment of accountability for individual program planning and implementation, and identifies the "trade offs" possible in a time frame should the need arise. The master plan takes shape from the overall goals as well as from the specific goals for the time period that it covers. Thus it gives direction to the staff development efforts. For example, if one of the goals is related to development of leadership skills for head nurses, the master plan would include the learning offerings planned for attaining this goal. A time frame of a year is usually followed in master planning; however, a shorter time period may be more feasible within certain settings. The development of the master plan is followed by specific plans for each learning offering or for the individual blocks of time within the plan.

Specific learning offering plans

The aim of any learning offering plan is to provide a record of the decisions made concerning the offering. This plan may include the objectives; the major topics within the content area; the time and length of the offering; correlation with other offerings; the media, materials, and teaching staff; the process strategies; any available alternative learning systems; and the evaluation process. Teaching plans are discussed further in Chapter 8.

Annual report

The annual report is designed to inform the nursing and agency administration of the staff development efforts during the past year and the prospects for the future. The content is prepared keeping in mind that the reader seeks understanding from it. In acquiring a relevant data base for the report, an outline is helpful. This may be drafted by the agency, the nursing department, or the staff development administrator. Although all staff development educators may submit an annual report of their particular activities, the annual report of staff development is prepared by the administrative staff development educator. Agreement on the "thrust" of the information and future plans is advisable.

In essence, an annual report is a "view" of the status of the programs, activities, and results obtained, with a projection into the future. Major content areas may include learning offerings, projects, research efforts, and a report on the year's accomplishments in relation to goals and staff activities. Staff activities may include service on committees and service given to special projects as well as professional and community activities. Major problems affecting the staff development efforts should be cited because these may have an effect on any aspect of the program or may influence effective utilization of the staff. New programs initiated in other areas that have had an impact on staff development should be noted. Trends that are influencing or will be influencing future programming also are cited. A timetable for input and for submitting annual reports should be set. A data base for self-renewal efforts is an important aspect of the design of the annual report.

Interim reports

Monthly or quarterly reports on activities may be required in some agencies in addition to an annual report. Having such data and reviewing it on a regular basis can provide an overall view of the status of the learning offerings and may be a critical factor in management decisions if a management style exists where this kind of information is not reviewed on a continuing basis. Review and analysis of the information in any regular reporting mechanism can assist in the defining and resolving of problem areas on both a staff and individual level.

Individual and group employee records

Verification of an employee's attendance at a learning offering should be documented and kept on file. This evidence is useful for the agency with regard to accreditation standards, legal requirements in selected offerings, and promotion purposes. An attendance record may be kept as part of an individual or group record.

An achievement record provides information about the level of competency reached in a particular learning offering. It may be given in the form of a certificate and is usually incorporated in the employee's personnel file.

Participation in continuing education activities outside the agency should be documented in a similar fashion. In some agencies a questionnaire is used for obtaining information to update the individual employee's record.

A checklist or a skills inventory is another type of individual employee record. The skills inventory and the application form should complement each other in terms of a data base. The information from these records is more accessible if it can be programmed on a computer.

Class records also comprise a data base for the educator's use. Such records usually include a satisfactory or unsatisfactory rating based on evidence of knowledge or of performance; what modules an employee needs to take in a selected course may be recorded. Before a person is given responsibility it must be determined whether or not that individual possesses the knowledge and ability needed to fulfill the responsibility. Records of learning offerings should be maintained to determine if the participant meets the standards of the program.

Statistical records

The purpose of statistical data is to project future needs, to review past efforts, and to show tangible output. The statistics may be in terms of attendance, categories of personnel, learning offerings (perhaps by numbers), and time. This data also may serve other purposes, including the comparison of assets with needs.

Evaluation records

Evaluation records provide information about the successes and failures of the learners, the individual offerings, and the total effort. It is necessary to maintain some records of evaluation, which is discussed in greater detail in Chapter 10.

Budget reports

As discussed previously, the budgetary format is usually provided by the agency. For the sake of comparison, it is important to keep these files for several years. The preceding budget should be most useful in projecting the next; even earlier budgets may provide useful information.

Statements on professional standards

Within the health team, as roles and relationships change, professional organizations have begun to issue statements or standards of practice in an effort to clarify the role of the practitioners of that profession. In the absence of specific laws, these statements or standards have legal ramifications. Therefore it is imperative for the staff development educator to maintain an up-to-date file of such statements or standards. When two or more professional groups within an agency develop a particular statement, it should be in accordance with the laws, statements, or standards governing the professions involved. Copies of these agency statements should be retained.

SUMMARY

Throughout this chapter emphasis has been placed on the need to organize an effective and efficient program of staff development to facilitate the administration of the total effort and to meet the learning needs within the agency. Because organization of staff development is based on the philosophy and goals of the agency, variances in organizational patterns exist among agencies. Additionally, how staff development is administered may vary, depending on the organizational structure and available resources.

Periodic review of the effectiveness of staff development organization needs to be made in terms of ever-changing situations. No matter what approach is used, it must be flexible, adaptable, and allow for the effective implementation of learning systems.

REFERENCES

1. Joint Commission for Accreditation of Hospitals: Accreditation manual, Chicago, 1970, The Commission.
2. American Nurses' Association: Standards for nursing services, Kansas City, Mo., 1973, The Association.
3. American Nurses' Association: Avenues for continued learning, Kansas City, Mo., 1967, The Association.
4. Davis, R. C.: Planning human resource development, Chicago, 1966, Rand McNally & Co.
5. Boutwell, C. E.: Differentiated staffing as a component in a systematic change process, Educ. Technol. **12:**20, Aug. 1972.

BIBLIOGRAPHY

Alexander, E. L.: Nursing administration in the hospital health care system, St. Louis, 1972, The C. V. Mosby Co.

Bennis, W. G.: Organization development: its nature, origin, and prospects, Reading, Mass., 1969, Addison-Wesley Publishing Co., Inc.

Dale, E.: Organization, New York, 1967, American Management Association, Inc.

Fry, W. F., and Lauer, J.: The planning team: why include nursing membership, J. Nurs. Admin. **2**(5):70, 1972.

Ganong, W. L., and Ganong, J. M.: Reducing organizational conflict through working committees, J. Nurs. Admin. **1**(1):12. 1972.

Knowles, M. S.: The modern practice of adult education, New York, 1970, Association Press.

March, J. J.: Handbook of organization, Chicago, 1965, Rand McNally & Co.

Marciniszyn, C.: Decentralization of nursing service, J. Nurs. Admin. **1**(4):17, 1971.

Miller, D. J.: Administration for the patient, Am. J. Nurs. **65:**114, 1965.

National League for Nursing: A self-evaluation guide for nursing services in hospitals and related institutions, New York, 1967, Council of Hospital and Related Institutional Nursing Services.

Stowe, R. A.: The critical issue in instructional development, Audiovis. Instr. **16:**8, Dec., 1971.

6

Philosophy, purpose and goals: option or necessity?

The discovery of what is true and practice of that which is good are the two most important objects of philosophy.

VOLTAIRE

A philosophy can be defined very simply as what one values or believes. All individuals have a personal philosophy that motivates their actions and determines how they manage their lives. Likewise, a philosophy of staff development is a statement of beliefs that serves as a guideline for determining a program of staff development. These beliefs form the basis for developing definitions, objectives, content, and methods of instruction.

This description seems clear and logical; yet in talking with others about improving the effectiveness of an existing staff development program or implementing a new program, it is not unusual to find lack of support for a written philosophy or a negative reaction to an already existing written statement. There seems to be a feeling that giving written expression to beliefs about staff development is an insurmountable task or an academic exercise. Some individuals involved in staff development have been exposed to philosophies in their educational programs or positions in nursing that have no apparent relationship to the curriculum or mission of the agency and that are written in professional jargon not easily understood or translatable into action. Others have worked in an environment where no written philosophy of nursing exists and therefore have no model to follow. Moore suggests that the development of such statements is a way of avoiding self-examination.

This tendency to make use of pot-boiler statements culled from the folklore of nursing does serve a purpose of sorts; it protects nurses from looking at the realities of their jobs and evaluating their own activities. If the philosophy, purpose and objectives are stated in sufficiently non-functional terms, the ideas in question cannot be used as a basis for checking whether activities are in line with what one says she believes and is trying to achieve. The avoidance of self-examination is not restricted to nurses; we share it with the rest of humanity.°

A well-written philosophy stated in meaningful, operational terms is a necessity for planning, organizing, implementing, and evaluating a staff development program. It serves as a guide and provides direction to those responsible for program planning. Without it, the program is like a ship without a rudder—sailing in all different directions, but never achieving the main purpose or goal.

In an article concerning continuing education, Coye highlights this very point in her discussion of the need for a written philosophy.

> I would recommend that a good place to start is to sit down alone or with your staff and consciously identify what you believe about continuing education and to put

°Moore, M. A.: Philosophy, purpose and objectives: why do we have them? J. Nurs. Admin. 1(3):9, 1971.

55

Table 6-1. Elements of a philosophy

Elements	Philosophical statements
Statement denoting congruence with the philosophy of nursing	The philosophy of staff development is based on the philosophy of nursing that identifies its obligation to provide nursing care to long-term patients and facilities for the education of students of nursing.
Categories of nursing personnel involved in providing nursing care	The role expectations delineated for the various types of nursing personnel are used as a basis for orientation and continuing education.
Obligation of the agency for providing learning opportunities	With the rapid advance in technologies resulting in changing practices of patient care, it is imperative that opportunities be provided for all employees to maintain and improve their individual practice, which additionally may assist in attainment of job satisfaction.
Responsibility of the employees for their own continuing learning	The employees are expected to identify and seek opportunities for learning based on their own individual needs.
Recognition of learners as adults	The learners in staff development are adults; therefore the concepts of adult learning are utilized in program planning.
Responsibility for identification of learning needs and planning to meet these needs	The responsibility for identifying learning needs, providing opportunities for meeting these needs, and evaluating the effectiveness of learning activities lies with the learners and their immediate superiors. Persons assigned to staff development positions provide supporting services to the clinical personnel and work in a collaborative relationship to assist the staff in becoming more knowledgeable and competent in fulfilling role expectations.
Definition of staff development	Staff development includes both formal and informal learning opportunities taking place within and outside the agency.
Purpose of staff development	The major purpose of staff development is change in behavior resulting in improved patient care through increased knowledge, understanding, skill, and changing attitudes.
Organization of staff development	Development of personnel is best accomplished through provision of learning opportunities in the immediate clinical environment. High value is placed on clinical knowledge and competence; therefore priority in programming is given to clinical content pertinent to the patient population and provision made for personnel to work with clinically competent role models.

Table 6-1. Elements of a philosophy—cont'd

Elements	Philosophical statements
Components of the program	The two main components of staff development are orientation and continuing education. Skill training and leadership development are integral parts of both.
Effecting planned change	Staff development assists the employees in adapting to new demands or needs of the nursing service or agency

these beliefs into a statement of philosophy about the matter. It took me a long time to learn how valuable this process can be. As I look back, I find my beliefs on this subject have changed many times over the past years, as I'm sure yours have or will. Until I faced these facts, for all the efforts I extended under the name of continuing education, I had great difficulty observing much evidence that patients were better cared for because of anything I was doing. Out of this realization, I developed a new list of beliefs around which the new goals for my present program are reorganized.°

DEVELOPING A PHILOSOPHY

If staff development programming is to have an influence on the improvement of patient care, it must be an integral part of the organization of the nursing service. Therefore developing the philosophy is a joint endeavor between staff development personnel and clinical personnel. A staff development person may provide the leadership but not to the extent of excluding the ideas of those most closely involved in providing nursing care to patients. A philosophy developed by staff development personnel alone and distributed to the clinical services is a useless tool. Unfortunately this often happens and results in a centralized program with little effect on change in behavior.

One approach is for the staff development

°Coye, D. H.: What is continuing education in nursing service? Supervisor Nurse 1(11):37, 1970.

personnel first to develop the basic concepts and then to utilize the clinical personnel as reactors. For example, a group of head nurses or selected personnel from various units could serve as a reaction group, depending on the individual setting. The important point here is that persons involved directly in nursing practice should provide input.

Another approach, probably the most effective, is to form a small work group with representatives from the clinical services and staff development. Active involvement by both groups provides (1) the opportunity for discussions of ideas and beliefs from two frames of reference and (2) greater commitment on the part of clinical personnel because they have had a role in the formulation of statements of belief. This approach benefits the agency because more persons are directly involved with the process, the clinical personnel gain a better understanding of the benefits of staff development, and the staff development educator receives a clearer picture of the nursing practice situation.

No matter which approach is used in developing the philosophy, some of the questions that must be considered are the following:

- What is the philosophy of the agency and nursing service?
- Why is staff development necessary?
- What is the major purpose?
- Whose responsibility is it—the agency's, the individual's, or both?
- What is staff development and what does it include?

• Who is responsible for identifying learning needs and providing for learning opportunities?

The philosophy of staff development must be consistent with the purposes of the agency and the philosophy of nursing. Therefore in developing a philosophy, the first step is to become familiar with the specific purpose of the agency and the ways in which the philosophy of nursing reflects these purposes. In the event that no written nursing philosophy exists, it is still proper to develop a staff development philosophy. However, beliefs about the type of patient services provided (acute, long-term, etc.), the expectations of nursing personnel, and the commitments of the department to the nursing personnel must be determined. These areas of concern are basic to the content of a staff development philosophy. Little and Carnevali[1] cite several philosophies of nursing service. Those persons developing or revising a philosophy of nursing service may find this a useful reference.

Before putting anything in writing, the literature should be explored to obtain ideas that will be helpful in answering the many questions that will arise. In addition, terms need to be defined early in the process so that all persons involved are working with the same frame of reference. For example, what is continuing education versus staff development or in-service education? What is leadership development? Does it differ from management development? A review of the current literature demonstrates little concensus in the answers to these questions. The participants will need to determine what definition is appropriate for their particular setting. This point cannot be stressed enough, since a great deal of time can be wasted by lack of a common understanding of terminology.

Before submitting a final draft to an approving body or individual, it is useful to obtain the reactions of others in the nursing service. This not only allows for more active involvement in the formulation but also may facilitate implementation, as the person most affected by the proposal will have had the opportunity to read it and make suggestions for its revision. In such circumstances the philosophy is more likely to be accepted and utilized as a guide in staff development programming by all the personnel. Since this is the major objective in developing a written philosophy, it is well worth the effort to involve as many persons in its development as is practical and reasonable.

ELEMENTS OF A PHILOSOPHY

There are several elements that are essential in a philosophy of staff development. The philosophical statement or beliefs related to these elements will vary with each agency. Therefore the examples cited in Table 6-1 are only guidelines for those embarking on the project of putting in writing what they believe.

As mentioned previously, the philosophy must reflect the purposes of the agency and the nursing service. There is no *one* philosophy that will meet the needs of all agencies. As seen in Exhibits B and E in the Appendix, philosophies in similar institutions differ in accordance with the agency, nursing philosophies, and organization.

DELINEATING THE PURPOSE

When the philosophy is completed, a review of the beliefs should indicate not only what staff development entails but why it is necessary. Price,[2] in a review of literature, found minor differences in definitions of in-service education. Today the purpose and definition of staff development in nursing seem to be more controversial. Some individuals support the concept that staff development programming includes only those learning experiences planned within the agency. This concept is narrow in scope and does not support the utilization of learning opportunities planned by professional and community organizations, universities, and colleges as a part of staff development.

In delineating a purpose of staff development, serious consideration needs to be given to what the agency can and will support. The

Table 6-2. Examples of developing goals and objectives from philosophical statements

Example 1

Philosophical statement	Development of personnel is best accomplished through provision of learning opportunities in the immediate clinical environment. High value is placed on clinical knowledge and competence; therefore priority in programming is given to clinical content pertinent to the patient population and provision made for personnel to work with clinically competent role models.
Goal	Facilitate the concept of decentralized staff development by providing opportunities for learning in the immediate clinical environment, with the major focus on the needs of a particular patient population and the personnel assigned to provide care for these patients.
General objective (orientation)	Acquire basic knowledge and skill in application of nursing practice policies and procedures necessary to provide safe nursing care specific to a particular patient population.
Specific objective (orientation for registered nurses)	Given the opportunity over a four-week period to administer nursing care to a group of orthopedic patients, the registered nurse assesses nursing care requirements and records them on the nursing care plan within the framework of the nursing practice policies and procedures specific to that patient population.

Example 2

Philosophical statement	The learners in staff development are adults; therefore the concepts of adult learning are utilized in program planning.
Goal	Create a climate for learning that will facilitate the teaching-learning process for both staff and students of nursing.
General objective (leadership development)	Apply concepts of andragogy in planning continuing education offerings in the clinical environment.
Specific objective (leadership development for registered nurses)	Given the opportunity to develop a teaching plan in a simulated setting, the registered nurse will be able to teach nurse assistants a new technique or procedure in the clinical environment utilizing the principles of andragogy.

following statement of purpose reflects the philosophy expressed in Table 6-1. *The purpose of staff development is (1) to promote improved patient care through support of educational activities that are directed toward change in behavior related to role expectations and (2) to facilitate the attainment of the individual's work-oriented goals.* Thus the purpose is a crystallization of the philosophy, giving meaning and direction to it.

DETERMINING THE GOALS AND OBJECTIVES

The overall goals of the staff development program are based on and are consistent with the staff development philosophy and purpose. They should be clearly stated but broad in nature. They give direction to the delineation of general objectives for each component of the overall program. Evaluation of their relevancy to the needs of the consumer and the learners is an ongoing process. (See Appendix, Exhibits C, D, and E.)

General objectives define expectations for change in behavior relative to a broad area or component of the total program. For example, there are certain basic behaviors inherent in the position or role expectations of the learner. The general objectives for each component form the basis for evaluation of the total staff development program.

Objectives developed for each offering within the component, such as orientation for registered nurses, are specific to the learning needs of the participants and are stated in terms of measurable change in behavior. The specific behaviors are congruent with the general objectives and provide direction for selection of course content, learning experiences, and evaluation of change in behavior.

The examples in Table 6-2 illustrate how the philosophy provides direction for the delineation of goals and objectives.

In summary, staff development goals are broad statements reflecting the major concepts in the philosophy. General objectives define expectations for change in behavior relative to a broad area or component of the total program. Specific objectives are statements of measurable behaviors expected as a result of a specific offering.[3]

REFERENCES

1. Little, D. E., and Carnevali, D. L.: Nursing care planning, Philadelphia, 1969, J. B. Lippincott Co.
2. Price, E. M.: Learning needs of registered nurses, New York, 1967, Teachers College Press.
3. Western Interstate Commission for Higher Education: Continuing education in nursing, Boulder, Colo., 1969, The Commission.

BIBLIOGRAPHY

Alexander, E. L.: Nursing administration in the hospital health care system, St. Louis, 1972, The C. V. Mosby Co.

American Nurses' Association: Statement of beliefs on inservice education and functions and qualifications for inservice educators, Kansas City, Mo., 1966, The Association.

Cooper, S. S., and Hornback, M. S.: Continuing nursing education, New York, 1973, McGraw-Hill Book Co.

Coye, D. H.: What is continuing education in nursing service? Supervisor Nurse 1(11):36, 1970.

Houle, C. O.: The design of education, San Francisco, 1972, Jossey-Bass, Inc., Publishers.

MacPhail, J.: An experiment in nursing: planning, implementing and assessing planned change, Cleveland, 1972, The Press of Case Western Reserve University.

Moore, M. A.: Philosophy, purpose and objectives: why do we have them? J. Nurs. Admin. 1(3):9, 1971.

Tobin, H. M., and Wengerd, J. S.: What makes a staff development program work? Am. J. Nurs. 71:940, 1971.

Tyler, R. W.: Basic principles of curriculum and instruction, Chicago, 1949, University of Chicago Press.

7

Identifying learning needs

It is impossible for anyone to begin to learn what he thinks he already knows.

EPICTETUS

Nurses are continually talking about "meeting patient needs." This is a very broad term and it is doubtful that even under the best circumstances the patient's total needs are met. The patient has basic human needs that may not have a direct relationship to his present illness but indirectly may affect his recovery. For example, a chronic alcoholic hospitalized for three days due to an injured foot obviously has psychological and social needs other than those directly related to his injury; the time factor dictates that these needs will not be met in this brief period. He may be observed for delirium tremens and referrals may be made regarding his alcoholic status, but the needs that are met are those specific to nursing care requirements related to his injured foot. In this situation the patient's total needs have not been met.

In the same way, the staff development educator must be concerned with and understand the influence of basic human needs on the teaching-learning process as discussed in Chapter 4. For example, employees low in seniority with families to support most likely will find it difficult to concentrate on learning on a day that restrictions in the personnel budget are announced. In addition, the educator must be cognizant of organizational and societal factors and changes that influence learning needs, as discussed in Chapters 5 and 11. Needs for change in health care systems greatly influence the roles of all health workers. For example, the introduction of the nurse clinician into the nursing service has affected the organizational structure and has, in many situations, been considered a threat by nursing personnel, particularly head nurses. Their ability to accept the nurse clinicians as resource persons in all probability will influence their capacity to learn from the nurse clinicians, even though they have a learning need. These forces exist in any setting, and the identification of learning needs should take into account the extenuating circumstances that influence the learner's ability to perform.

WHAT IS A LEARNING NEED?

Webster's dictionary defines a need as something useful, required, or desired that is lacking or a condition in which there is a deficiency of something. The latter definition as applied to learning needs is questioned by Mager and Pipe.[1] They prefer to use the word "discrepancy," pointing out that discrepancy means only that there is a difference between what is and what is desired, whereas the use of the term "deficiency" implies that the discrepancy is bad or unacceptable. It is like using the term "gap" to describe the difference between what is taught in basic nursing programs and what is expected of the beginning nursing practitioner. The value judgment made by nursing educators about this term is much different than that made by nursing service personnel. Therefore in identifying learning needs, one must be careful not to jump to conclusions before analyzing the situation.

Just because a discrepancy exists does not mean there is always a need for an educational activity. The discrepancy may be a symptom rather than the real learning need. Staff development often is considered to be the "panacea for all ills," when, indeed, the problem may be a need for modification or change in the environment or standard of care rather than a learning need. In analyzing a discrepancy between what a group of nurses are being taught and what is done in actual practice, it may be found that the policy or procedure being taught is in need of change rather than the performance of the nurses. For example, there may be a standing order in the maternity nursing service that patients are to be catheterized eight hours following delivery if they have not voided. The nurses ignore the standing order and use judgment based on clinical data as to whether or not and when the patients need catheterizing. After investigating the situation, action is taken to discontinue the standing order, and broad policies are developed as guidelines. In another situation, nurses may know how to develop written nursing care plans, but little value is placed on this skill by the leadership personnel. Although developing written nursing care plans is delineated in the role expectations and the nurses have demonstrated satisfactory performance previously, few plans probably will be developed without an accountability and reward system for the nurses. In this case a learning need exists both on the part of the leadership personnel and the staff nurses to meet their role expectations regarding nursing care plans.

In still another situation, patients respond on their questionnaires that their bed linen is not being changed as frequently as it should be. They indicate that the staff does not want to take time to change the linen. In investigating the situation, it is found that a long-standing problem of the laundry not sending enough linen has become worse, and even

though this has been reported, no action has been taken to correct it. An organizational need exists here, not a learning need.

Learning needs are not always so easy to identify as those indicated in the preceding examples. A staff development educator needs to analyze each situation to be certain where the discrepancy lies.

In summary, for the purposes of this discussion a learning need is described as the discrepancy between what employees know and can do and what they need to learn to carry out role expectations or to prepare for additional responsibility.

APPROACHES TO IDENTIFYING NEEDS

The job of identifying learning needs would be a simple one if every employee within a job classification brought the same knowledge, skills, and attitudes to the position. In years past, nurses were a more homogeneous group in relation to their practice skills than they are today. As pointed out by Tobin and Wengerd:

> . . . social forces—the youth movement, student unrest, and changes in educational programs—influence young nurses today just as they affect other young people. New graduates come with varied educational preparation and specific expectations. They are more vocal and more critical of the establishment. Moreover, variations within the three types of nursing programs make it even more difficult to identify common learning needs of new graduates that a centralized program can meet. These factors affect registered nurses' attitudes toward learning and should influence the approach to teaching.[°]

Because each nurse, as well as other employees, differs in knowledge, skills, and attitudes, the task of finding out just what they need to learn in order to fulfill their specific role expectations is very complex. As the employees develop in their role identification, needs for continued individual learning as well

°Tobin, H., and Wengerd, J.: What makes a staff development program work? Am. J. Nurs. 71:940, 1971.

as the needs of groups add to the complexity of the situation.

Before the staff development process can begin, role expectations, policies, and procedures must be developed, as seen in Fig. 1-2, p. 5. If there is no agreement on what is expected and how well it is to be done, there can be little agreement in the identification of discrepancies that indicate learning needs or in the subsequent programming necessary to develop the personnel. The development of job standards is not the primary role of the staff development educator; it belongs to those in the clinical service and the consumers of health care. The educator has a participative role and may act as the facilitator by serving as the group leader delegated to accomplish the task. This part of the process is difficult, can be very frustrating, and may result in a tendency to accept the existing conditions while ignoring the problems. Observation of individual performances with subsequent interviews will most likely verify that misunderstandings do exist. Unless such a situation is ameliorated, any change in behavior that approaches the desired goals will be by happenstance. In order to measure improvement, there must be standards against which to measure change. Therefore, although it would be easier to omit this first step, it must be undertaken if an effective program is to be developed.

In carrying out a needs analysis, the personal goals and needs of the individuals and the goals and needs of the organization must be integrated in order to facilitate attainment of both. A staff development educator must be familiar with a variety of means to identify each employee's needs and the needs of the organization in order to plan meaningful learning offerings.

For the purposes of this book, identification of needs is divided into four areas: (1) observation of personnel performance, (2) verbal and written communication with and from personnel, (3) analysis of records and reports, and (4) changes within and outside the agency.

Observation of performance

Direct observation of work performance is probably the best method of identifying learning needs. However, because it is not possible for a staff development educator to observe everyone at all times, others in leadership positions (supervisors, head nurses, team leaders, etc.) must be relied on to assist in collecting these data. It is crucial, however, that the educator undertake some direct observation in the clinical services. Depending on the organization, there are several ways in which this can be accomplished. Whatever the approach, it is important that the method be carefully planned and purposeful and not implemented in an arbitrary fashion.

Staff development educators working directly in the clinical area with personnel have a golden opportunity to observe the performance of individuals as well as the working relationships among people. Although the primary reason for being there may be supervision of a group of new nurse assistants, orientation of a licensed practical nurse, or working with registered nurses in their team leader or primary nurse° roles, the opportunity exists to make general observations of others in the immediate environment. In order to collect meaningful data, the purpose of these observations must be defined.

Attending change-of-shift reports and conferences, reviewing nursing care plans, observing how personnel interact and communicate with patients (both verbally and nonverbally) and with each other, as well as observing clinical skills will provide valuable data regarding learning needs. However, it is important to remember that observations must be made over a period of time before valid judgments can be made concerning the learning needs of an individual, a classification of employees, or the entire unit staff. If observations are made that indicate the immediate safety of the patient is endangered, intervention measures rather than data collection

°Primary nurse is used in terms of the role as defined by Manthey (see bibliography).

have priority. As discussed earlier, what is observed may be a symptom of an organizational problem that needs to be corrected before the symptom can be alleviated.

Although not so meaningful, the staff development educator might also observe performance by making regular rounds to the clinical areas on all tours of duty, either alone or with the supervisor or head nurse. How these rounds are approached depends on the relationship with the clinical personnel. If the educator is readily visible every day and is accepted as a "helping person," the need to be accompanied by the supervisor or head nurse will be lessened. However, on occasions it can be useful to have the head nurses or supervisors present so that they can comment on needs at the time the observations are made. In addition, they will usually provide important feedback regarding their observations of personnel performance following staff development activities. If the educator appears only occasionally, unless a trusting relationship has been established in other ways, it most likely will be appropriate to request the company of the supervisor or head nurse. In either case, the purpose for making these rounds needs to be understood by the personnel if they are to cooperate in identifying learning needs. In order to collect meaningful data, the objectives should be defined. It is often helpful to develop a form for recording observations in the various areas. This approach helps in tabulating and analyzing the data. Following are but a few of the many areas of observations that might be recorded.

- Are the registered nurses involved in direct patient care, or are they observed most frequently in the nurses' station?
- Are all personnel occupied, or do some seem unusually busy and others often not occupied?
- Are the verbal and nonverbal communications conducive to effective working relations—both between nursing personnel and other hospital personnel?
- Do patients appear well-cared for; that is, are comfort measures, safety measures, and interaction between staff and patients appropriate?

- Are nursing care techniques carried out in a safe and effective manner?
- Are nursing care plans developed and, if so, are they utilized as a basis for giving nursing care?

The most obvious opportunity for direct observation by the staff development educator occurs while working directly with an individual or group in the clinical setting or in the classroom. The observations made relate directly to the learning needs of these persons but can also serve as a basis for program revision when similar needs are identified with several individuals and groups over a period of time. For example, it might be observed that the last four groups of registered nurses in a leadership development workshop have had difficulty in applying the concepts of the evaluation process, even though they have attended previous workshops on this subject. Therefore an analysis of the situation is indicated that includes interviewing the supervisors and head nurses to determine the nurses' role in evaluating the performance of other personnel. It may be found that they have not been expected to utilize the content offered, or if there was this expectation, that they were unable to fulfill it effectively. In either case, a learning need exists that necessitates some change in programming. Perhaps the content needs to be expanded, the sequence of learning offerings changed, or conferences held so leadership personnel can discuss the accountability of staff.

Verbal and written communication

Verbal communication. Both formal and informal communication with personnel are important sources of identifying needs. An informal discussion with personnel, for example, over a cup of coffee, may reveal a misunderstanding or lack of acceptance of a recent change in policy, a problem regarding assignments within a certain group of workers, or the need for more definite guidelines and instruction regarding a new piece of equipment or treatment procedure. Attendance at change-of-shift reports or team conferences may indicate a lack of understanding of a certain patient population or a need for assistance in organizing or making priority judgments about the needs of patients. As a staff development educator, it is necessary to seek out frequent, informal contacts with all kinds of nursing personnel in order to identify many "grass roots" learning needs.

Interaction with personnel at formal staff development programs such as workshops and conferences can also provide a ready source of data to help in determining needs. Participating in informal discussions at breaktime or following the offering, listening to the contributions of individuals, and evaluating their ability to attain the objectives will usually provide indicators of other learning needs. For example, at a workshop for head nurses on the group process it may be seen that they needed such knowledge earlier in their careers in order to identify and work effectively with the different groups on their units. In another situation the objective may be group identification of a problem or determination of alternative solutions to it; however, group members may be unable to get to this point because of difficulty in identifying the "real" problem itself. The inability of the group to identify the problem or determine alternate solutions indicates that the educator needs to change the focus of the objectives at that particular time.

There are some personnel or groups of personnel who are able to identify and articulate their own learning needs. For example, a group of registered nurses and licensed practical nurses may request a review of care for orthopedic patients in traction, since there has been an overflow on the orthopedic floor and these patients have been assigned to their unit. In another example a nurse on a pediatric unit may indicate a limited background in caring for children with cystic fibrosis and request assistance in planning nursing care for these patients.

On occasion it is appropriate to schedule formal interviews with leadership personnel and unit personnel to identify learning needs.

This can be done on a group basis, an individual basis, or both. For example, in revising an orientation program it may be desirable to schedule meetings with groups of supervisors, head nurses, and a representative group of other nursing personnel. In order to collect relevant data, the staff development educator should structure an interview guide or at least have in mind the kinds of questions to be asked. The subsequent analysis of data will then take place within a common framework and decision making will be facilitated. Some of the questions that might be asked include the following: (1) Have changes in role expectations and approaches to patient care occurred? (2) Do these changes have implications for revision of content or methods of teaching? (3) Do they indicate a need to decentralize some of the content now being taught centrally or vice versa? (4) Is there coordination between the centralized and decentralized teaching efforts?

It might be that feedback in leadership workshops for staff nurses indicates that nurse assistants do not understand the team nursing concept. Formal interviews might be scheduled with groups of nurse assistants to explore their understanding as well as with head nurses to identify their understanding of both nurse assistants and staff nurses. What is "heard" may indicate the need for change in teaching methods or for a more refined delineation of guidelines for team nursing in the particular setting.

Another source of communication is a staff development committee serving in either an advisory or planning capacity, depending on the particular setting. A major function of these committees is to identify learning needs. If the committee is to be an effective and reliable resource, it should be comprised of persons in various positions and specialties. Members should be chosen from among those who are keenly interested in the purpose of the committee and who are skilled in leadership.

Entrance interviews can provide a data base for orientation of individuals as well as for groups. In addition, exit interviews can elicit valuable information related to learning needs. The attainment of this information will depend mainly on the interviewer's skill in providing a climate that is conducive to an open airing of views. Analyzing data from these interviews over a period of time may indicate several areas of learning needs, particularly if turnover rates are high. In a study of baccalaureate nurses working in medical centers, Kramer and Baker[2] found that there was conflict between what the graduates perceived as their professional role and how that role was defined by the bureaucratic structure.

Being able to determine the individuals' needs (including learning needs) as well as the organizational needs may result in retaining the individual within the service. If only the organizational needs are considered, the individual may be motivated to seek other employment or leave nursing altogether. Face-to-face communication has the advantage of providing an opportunity for employees to express their opinions and suggestions openly and honestly, assuming that a climate exists in which they feel free to do so. They must feel that they are being listened to without being judged. One of the skills necessary in sorting out the real learning needs from symptoms is the ability to listen with understanding. This skill must be cultivated if learning needs data are to be collected through verbal communication. Too often we are prone to hear only what we want to hear because it is easier that way. If we really "listen," we may find that there are learning needs to be met that seem almost overwhelming. For example, it may be apparent after several interviews (both formal and informal) that a major learning need of young graduates is the ability to hold other personnel accountable for fulfilling their role expectations. If 50% of the staff have been out of a basic nursing program for less than one year, this fact alone can be staggering but not insurmountable.

Written communication. There are several approaches to collecting written information about learning needs and some examples are

(1) questionnaires, (2) skill inventories, (3) slip technique, (4) pretests and post-tests, and (5) performance appraisals. A brief description of these tools follows. For more specific information regarding their construction and use, refer to the bibliography.

Questionnaires. When it is possible to establish a clear, trusting relationship through frequent interaction with staff, the need to use questionnaires is lessened. However, when many people are involved, it may be the only means to reach all personnel in a short period of time. In addition, unlike face-to-face contact, the use of questionnaires allows for anonymity. An important factor to consider is the construction of the questionnaire. Assistance may be needed from someone skilled in the development of such tools if reliable data are to be collected. Knowles[3] cautions also that this technique should be used only if the results are going to be given to those who took the time to complete the questionnaire. Failure to do this will result in limited responses to future questionnaires.

In analyzing data from questionnaires, it should be remembered that what the employees indicate as learning needs are not always congruent with organizational needs. The staff development educator must try to satisfy both needs while focusing on programming that is in the best interest of the consumers. For example, the results of a questionnaire may indicate a high interest in a discussion on human sexuality, while direct observation of performance has indicated a need for greater understanding of fluid and electrolyte balance. Thus there is a need to have knowledge of both, but because of the acuity of patients within the hospital setting, the more urgent learning need probably relates to the knowledge of fluid and electrolyte balance. Priorities in programming need to be established. However, because the personnel were interested enough to express their learning need, every effort should be made to provide a discussion on human sexuality.

There are several approaches to constructing questionnaires. The open-ended question allows for greater freedom of response but is difficult to tabulate, while checklists or forced response–type questions lend themselves more readily to analysis. No matter what type of questionnaire is used, it is important that it be clear and concise. Often one's own experience with lengthy and unclear questionnaires is an invaluable guide in the attempt to achieve clarity. As suggested before, assistance should be sought from someone skilled in developing such tools and they should be tested before distribution to a large number of people.

Skill inventories. A skill inventory can be a useful tool in identifying the learning needs of individuals as well as groups. Usually the specified skills are based on the role expectations for a particular job classification and are stated in a "how to" form such as "how to make a bed" or "how to make out an assignment." Generally a three-point code is used, signifying the need for complete training, need for additional training, or no need because the performance is satisfactory. In addition, the information will provide a baseline for determining the size and number of classes to be scheduled as well as the number of educators needed to carry out the teaching program.

Slip technique.[4] The slip technique can be used to survey employees' perceptions of problems in the work environment and their ideas for solutions to these problems. For instance, head nurses may be having difficulty getting the registered nurses to develop written nursing care plans. In delineating the problem, the head nurses might pose the question "how can the head nurse assist the staff in developing written nursing care plans?" The staff would then write suggestions, each on the top of a separate slip of paper. A specific period of time (15 to 20 minutes) would be allowed for the expression of as many ideas as possible. Similar suggestions could then be grouped and evaluated as a basis for implementation.

This technique also can be used to identify the employees' perceptions of their own learning needs. In a sense the slip technique is like brainstorming, except that the suggestions are written and thus anonymous.

Pretests and post-tests. There are two major reasons for using pretests as a basis for identifying learning needs: (1) to determine whether or not individuals have knowledge and skills that are prerequisite to participating in a specific learning offering and (2) to determine what the participants already know based on the objectives of the offering. In the first situation an educator for a course in administration of medications for licensed practical nurses may wish to test the potential participants for computational skills. In the second situation the educator may wish to utilize the results of the pretest as a basis for modifying the teaching plan to meet more adequately the real needs of the learners.

Post-tests provide information regarding what the participants did or did not learn. The results can be used for providing remedial help to those who did not meet the objectives or for revising the teaching plan based on the readiness of the participants to learn.

Performance appraisals. Performance appraisals can be a valuable source of learning needs information. Involvement of the individuals in self-evaluation and determination of personal goals as a part of the appraisal process aids in the identification of their needs. Mutual goal setting by the individuals and their immediate superiors during the appraisal helps to clarify the roles of both in the learning process. A staff development educator also may be involved in assisting individuals to attain their goals of increased competency.

A review of written performance appraisals by staff development educators can serve two purposes: (1) to identify the learning needs of individuals and (2) to identify the needs of groups. For example, in reviewing the appraisals of registered nurses after six months of employment, it may be found that the majority of them have difficulty in evaluating the performance of their team members. Obviously the present teaching program is not meeting this need and either the expectation or the teaching method must be revised.

Analysis of records and reports

Although sometimes overlooked, records and reports can be helpful in identifying learning needs. However, records and reports often indicate symptoms of an organizational problem rather than a learning need. Therefore the data must be carefully analyzed before a teaching program is decided on.

Incident reports. Tabulation of incident reports can reveal valuable data that are useful to the staff development educator. For example, incident report data may indicate that several patients have fallen from their beds. In studying the situation, it may be found that the side rails are defective and sometimes slide down when the patients lean on them. Even though this fact has been reported frequently, no action has been taken to correct it. This is an organizational problem, not a learning need. In other situations, incident reports do reveal obvious learning needs. For example, reports might indicate an increase in falls from wheelchairs due to the staffs' negligence in locking the wheels when assisting patients to and from the chairs. Or there may be an increase in employees incurring "bad backs" because of improper body mechanics.

Patient questionnaires. Patient surveys may yield considerable data. It must be remembered that the consumers' perceptions of good nursing care may differ from those of the nursing staff. However, if several consumers indicate that the response to their calls for assistance involved long delays, it is probable that a learning need exists. The term "probable" is used because if there is inadequate staffing, an organizational need exists.

Turnover and absentee records. Turnover and absentee records may indicate a failure to provide adequate learning experiences. Employees may become disenchanted with an environment that does not provide them with adequate guidance to fulfill their role expectations and opportunities for development.

Statistical records. Records of breakage and maintenance repair may indicate that staff members are using equipment improperly or lack an appreciation of economy. Planning learning offerings using this kind of data as well as original cost data can at times have an influence on the staff's attitude toward proper utilization and economy.

Employment applications. Employment applications and profiles of individual employees can provide pertinent information regarding educational backgrounds and experiences. The data from applications is particularly useful in planning for individual orientation. For example, a plan for the orientation of a group of registered nurses with several years' experience may differ considerably from one for newly graduated nurses who have not yet taken their state boards. In addition, it is appropriate to utilize basic educational preparation of new graduates as a basis for planning leadership development offerings because of the differences in the knowledge they bring to the position.

Annual reports. Annual reports should contain information that can be utilized in determining short- and long-range goals for the total staff development effort as well as for specific offerings. The report may provide justification for recommendations in the budget that create new learning needs. For example, the budgetary support of a new hemodialysis unit may include funding for a program to prepare the personnel necessary for the unit's function.

Changes within and outside the agency

A staff development educator must be alert to potential changes in the roles of personnel, patient care programs, and facilities. In addition, societal changes such as women's rights and consumers demands for acceptable standards of health care and changes in basic preparatory programs in nursing are but a few of the many issues that affect staff development efforts. These issues are discussed in Chapter 11 but are mentioned here to emphasize that the staff development educator must be aware of these issues and changes as a basis for predicting learning needs of personnel.

Roles of personnel. In some instances there may be minor changes in role expectations of personnel, for instance, as brought about by the introduction of a new procedure. In this situation it is obvious that all personnel have a learning need. At other times the learning needs may be more complex; perhaps a complete change has been made in the organizational structure that affects everyone's role expectations. For example, introduction of the unit manager system entails a reorientation of nursing personnel (especially the registered nurses) to their role for providing direct patient care rather than such aspects as paperwork, equipment and supplies, and the physical environment. In this situation the identification of learning needs of groups as well as individuals becomes a major undertaking. Short- and long-range goals need to be defined as a basis for providing systematic learning experiences that will lead to the fulfillment of the new roles. The key attributes are patience and persistence.

Patient care programs. Changes in patient care programs may necessitate an extensive teaching program for those involved in caring for a specific patient population. For example, the introduction of the surgical procedure for total hip replacement has had a significant impact on the teaching programs for many different kinds of health workers such as physicians, nursing personnel, and physical therapists.

The advent of specialization has made it necessary that registered nurses be prepared to care for more specific patient populations such as those in coronary care, renal dialysis, and intensive care units. Planning to meet the learning needs of these nurses has been a major undertaking in some institutions.

Facilities. The reconstruction and addition of facilities have implications for increased orientation of personnel. For example, different patterns and approaches to organizing the staff at the unit level may be implemented because of a move into new facilities. Such reorganization might be mandatory if room arrangement, bed complement, and service facilities differ greatly from the previous facilities.

TRANSLATING NEEDS INTO ACTION

Once the needs are identified, it becomes necessary to establish priorities and to formulate general and specific objectives (see Fig. 1-2, p. 5).

Establishing priorities

In establishing priorities, it may be clear that one need is most dominant because it relates to input factors such as philosophy, standards, or goals. For example, one of the major goals of the department of nursing may be to implement the concept of self-evaluation and identification of personal goals. A needs survey indicates little understanding and application of this concept at present; therefore staff development offerings to assist personnel to understand and implement this concept would have high priority. Another goal might be to develop and implement standards of care for the various patient populations. If standards of care have not already been delineated, it is obvious that there will be a need for staff development offerings.

In addition to the input factors that influence priorities, the feasibility of meeting the needs must be considered. Economic factors, the abilities of personnel, and time factors must be taken into account. In other words, if there is no money to support the offering, if the qualifications of the personnel (both teachers and learners) preclude implementing the concept, or if the personnel cannot be released for staff development offerings, other priorities must be established.

In analyzing the needs, it is helpful to first categorize them. One approach is to list them as (1) needs related to the administration of the total program, (2) learning needs related to groups of personnel, or (3) learning needs related to individuals. Needs related to the administration of the program might be for additional library facilities, increased financial support, or an improved communications system between staff development and clinical personnel. Learning needs of groups might involve interviewing skills for registered nurses, nursing care to patients with aphasia for all personnel on a specific unit, or ambulating patients for a group of nurse assistants. Learning needs of individuals might include counseling techniques on the part of a supervisor or operation of a piece of equipment by a registered nurse.

Once the needs have been categorized and the priorities established, it is time to formulate objectives.

Formulating objectives

In recent years several books and articles have been published that discuss the formulation of objectives. The terminology used varies with each publication and includes behavioral objectives, performance objectives, instructional objectives, goals, etc. For our purposes, we have classified the objectives in terms of goals, general objectives, and specific objectives, as discussed in Chapter 6. At this point our emphasis will be on the development of specific objectives.

Although opinions vary as to the components and classification of objectives, Mager[5] and Bloom et al.[6] seem to be quoted most frequently. Mager identifies three components of an objective:

1. Terminal behavior—what the student will be able to do at the end of instruction
2. Conditions—the conditions under which the behavior will be expected to occur
3. Criteria—the level at which the individual will be expected to perform

Bloom et al. classify educational objectives into these parts:

1. Cognitive—those objectives concerned with knowledge, understanding, and intellectual skills such as problem solving

---

Cognitive domain

Objective: Following a discussion related to nurse-patient interaction, the registered nurse will identify in writing four phases of the nurse-patient relationship.

Components:

Condition	*Terminal behavior*	*Criteria*
Following a discussion related to nurse-patient interaction, the registered nurse	will identify in writing	four phases of the nurse-patient relationship

Affective domain

Objective: Given the opportunity to attend a leadership development workshop, the registered nurse demonstrates interest by participating in discussions and completing written assignments.

Components:

Condition	*Terminal behavior*	*Criteria*
Given the opportunity to attend a leadership development workshop, the registered nurse	demonstrates interest by	participating in discussions and completing written assignments

Psychomotor domain

Objective: After observing a demonstration of an intramuscular injection, the licensed practical nurse will return the demonstration in accordance with the established procedure.

Components:

Condition	*Terminal behavior*	*Criteria*
After observing a demonstration of an intramuscular injection, the licensed practical nurse	will return the demonstration	in accordance with the established procedure

2. Affective—those objectives concerned with feelings and emotions such as attitudes, values, appreciation, and interests
3. Psychomotor—objectives concerned with manipulative skills and coordination such as giving a bed bath

In the chart on p. 70, the objectives are categorized according to Bloom's taxonomy and identify Mager's three components.

In most instances only objectives related to the cognitive domain are formulated because they are easier to define. However, objectives related to the affective and psychomotor domain should not be neglected, as they are just as important to the learning needs of the individuals. Again, patience and persistence are needed to identify specific behavioral objectives related to changes in attitude.

The major aim then is to base objectives on specific behaviors so that change in behavior can be evaluated. In Chapter 10 the use of objectives in the evaluation process will be discussed. In addition, other uses of objectives include (1) determining relevant content and teaching methods, (2) communicating to learners what is expected, and (3) communicating with significant others the focus of the programming.

The preceding is but a brief overview of formulating objectives. The references and bibliography will provide further assistance.

REFERENCES

1. Mager, R. F., and Pipe, P.: Analyzing performance problems or "you really oughta wanna," Belmont, Calif., 1970, Fearon Publishers.
2. Kramer, M., and Baker, C.: The exodus: can we prevent it? J. Nurs. Admin. 1(3):15, 1971.
3. Knowles, M. S.: The modern practice of adult education, New York, 1970, Association Press.
4. Training and continuing education, Chicago, 1970, Hospital Research & Educational Trust.
5. Mager, R.: Preparing instructional objectives, Belmont, Calif., 1962, Fearon Publishers.
6. Bloom, B. S., et al., editors: Taxonomy of educational objectives: cognitive domain, New York, 1956, David McKay Co., Inc.

BIBLIOGRAPHY

Garrett, A. M.: Interviewing: its principles and methods, ed. 2 (revised by Elinor P. Zaki and Margaret M. Mangold), New York, 1972, Family Service ·Association of America.
Gronlund, N. E.: Stating behavioral objectives for classroom instruction, New York, 1970, Macmillan Publishing Co., Inc.
Gronlund, N. E.: Measurement and evaluation in teaching, New York, 1971, Macmillan Publishing Co., Inc.
Houle, C. O.: The design of education, San Francisco, 1972, Jossey-Bass, Inc., Publishers.
Kathwohl, D. R., et al.: Taxonomy of educational objectives: affective domain, New York, 1964, David McKay Co., Inc.
Lee, S. L.: The assessment, analysis and monitoring of educational needs, Educ. Technol. 13:28, April, 1973.
Litwack, L., Sakata, R., and Wykle, M.: Counseling, evaluation and student development in nursing education, Philadelphia, 1972, W. B. Saunders Co.
Mager, R. F.: Goal analysis, Belmont, Calif., 1972, Fearon Publishers.
Manthey, M.: Primary care is alive and well in the hospital, Am. J. Nurs. 73:83, 1973.
Medearis, N. D., and Popiel, E. S.: Guidelines for organizing inservice education, J. Nurs. Admin. 1(4):30, 1971
Miller, M. A.: Inservice education for hospital nursing personnel, New York, 1958, National League for Nursing.
Popham, W. J., and Baker, E. L.: Establishing instructional goals, Englewood Cliffs, N. J., 1970, Prentice-Hall, Inc.
Price, E. M.: Learning needs of registered nurses, New York, 1967, Teachers College Press.
Skinner, G.: What do practicing nurses want to know? Am. J. Nurs. 69:1662, 1969.
Tyler, R. W.: Basic principles of curriculum and instruction, Chicago, 1949, University of Chicago Press.
Western Interstate Commission for Higher Education: Continuing education in nursing, Boulder, Colo., 1969, The Commission.

8 Designing and implementing learning offerings

Out of the strain of doing,
Into the peace of the done.

JULIA WOODRUFF

After talking with other staff development educators and reviewing the literature, it is evident that the work of staff development is accomplished in a number of ways. Although there are various approaches to organizing learning experiences (that is, designation of components), the underlying framework for carrying out the functions of staff development is the same.

BASIC ELEMENTS

To accomplish the work of staff development, three broad areas must be considered—input, process, and output (see Fig. 1-2, p. 5). Input includes all the "givens" in a situation—individual learners, material resources (equipment and supplies), policies relating to staff development, educators available, goals of the agency, etc.

The process describes how the input is going to be handled. Climate setting and the planning mechanism "set the stage" for the process. The attitude toward staff development within the agency influences how the learners accept the offerings. For example, lack of commitment on the part of staff may reduce the motivation of new employees to adhere to standards. If the agency does not value education, there may be too little equipment and too few staff development educators. The attitude may affect how needs are identified and how plans are made.

The planning mechanism, as discussed in the previous chapters, involves many aspects.

Planning fosters a more organized, enduring effect than when little or no effort is made. The planning mechanism refers to the structure of the staff development effort. Six basic elements constitute the framework of the process phase.

Identify needs

As discussed in Chapter 7, identifying learning needs is the first step in meeting them. If the needs are not well defined, the offerings may not be appropriate. In settings where new personnel are employed frequently a major effort would be required for orientation. Thus orientation offerings would be organized accordingly. If an agency changes the way in which people within a given classification function, additional needs could be identified that might require major programming efforts. Identified needs must be analyzed to determine if they are relevant to the agency's goals and if they are amenable to staff development.

Formulate objectives

The designation of objectives for each offering provides a basis for evaluating the output. Additionally, it provides a basis for content specific to the objective. The objective is based on the identified needs and should be behaviorally oriented. When objectives are stated in terms of the behaviors expected, it is more likely that the learners will recognize whether or not they have met the expectations and thus may be more aware of their learning needs. For example, if the learners know they must be able to present three anecdotal records, identifying the who, what, when, where, how, and why factors, they will have the direction necessary to produce the desired information. Formulating objectives may lead to the identification of a group of related objectives, with the result that offerings emerge. Additionally, the objectives should imply toward whom the learning activity is directed and for what purpose. The grouping of objectives may lead to the formulation of some ideas about designing the components of staff development.

Define topics

The topics of staff development programs are based on the needs and objectives. At times they may be grouped together to form a course for a particular group of employees. Topics need to be limited to the specific objectives and focused on the defined need so that broad, nonspecific offerings are avoided. Adult learning principles influence how the topics are constructed. As stated in Chapter 3, the key concepts about how adults learn relate primarily to how the content of a program will be defined and organized. For example, although the identified need is very basic, a program related to it may require some detailed planning to allow for the individuals to express their own perceptions and relate the content to their own goals.

Resources influence how a topic will be dealt with. In planning a program as well as in designing the learning offerings, the available resources must be considered. For example, the number of available staff development educators may affect the approach to a topic. The setting may be one where clinical experts are available to supplement the efforts of the staff development educators. Although the setting may not have a particular piece of audiovisual equipment, it may be possible to design meaningful visual aid materials for the existing system. For example, if there is a videotape on a particular subject but the

agency does not have the basic system with which to show it, an overlay-type transparency may be made to supplement the basic discussion.

A third consideration is that of resources outside the agency. For example, if special nursing skills are needed in the postoperative care of total joint replacement patients, it should be determined whether a major medical center, a local college or university, or a professional association offers the desired course.

Another point to consider is the use of equipment that may be available to your agency. It may not be realistic for all agencies to spend a great deal on a self-instructional system that is limited to a particular clinical area such as coronary care. However, two or three area agencies with coronary care units may be able to share the equipment and educators of one agency or combine their efforts to develop a course that would be more effective than if each had acted alone.

As cited in Chapter 9, methodology often determines the design of the learning offering. For example, if the only facility available can be used for lectures only, it may be difficult to include small group discussions within a particular offering. However, there may be space on individual units that could be used for small group discussions. The larger group would reconvene in the major classroom.

Some topics lend themselves to discussion rather than to formal lecture; some lend themselves to role-playing and others do not. The facility and resources have to be analyzed to determine what methodology best meets the needs.

Generally speaking, the sequence of topics should proceed from general to specific and from simple to complex. Sequence refers to the process of building on existing knowledge and skills in order to develop more comprehensive abilities. Thus some agencies offer courses that are divided into two parts, with the expectation that in the intervening period of time the employees will be able to make practical use of the content learned in the first half of the course. One of the best known techniques of sequential learning is that of programmed instruction, whereby the basic concepts, the normal, expected findings, and finally the deviations from the normal are identified. The assumption is that learners will understand the abnormal and its causes once they recognize what is normal.

If a specific topic is covered in more than one offering, it is particularly important to be alert to attendance. People who have not attended the previous segments of a particular course may be lacking the knowledge and skills on which to build. Another factor to consider in sequence relates to adult learning needs. Adults often demand immediate application of what has been learned, and this fact should be considered in developing the sequence of topics. As pointed out earlier in this book, nurses frequently want to be involved clinically from the beginning of their employment.

If a course is presented in a series of sessions, each session should have defined objectives that represent a specific portion of the total course. In this way no learners are left "hanging" between sessions. In planning this way, it may be necessary to devote unequal blocks of time to the various segments. If this is understood in advance and the blocks are not too long, the learners should be able to plan their time accordingly.

When a course is segmented, group interaction must be considered. It is beneficial if the same people can attend each session so that the interaction benefits the learner.

Continuity, on the other hand, is a basic reinforcement mechanism whereby some particular point is constantly reiterated. For example, if one of the themes for the year relates to nursing care plans, this concept might be incorporated in patient-centered conferences or grand rounds. In orientation offerings, everything needs to be related to preparing the individual to function within a defined position. Again, continuity should meet the individuals' needs (which may be immediate) as well as prepare them to ful-

fill their role expectations at the end of orientation.

Design plan of learning experiences

This step involves the actual development of the program and includes the teaching plan and time schedule and staff assignment.

The teaching plan. All organized learning offerings should proceed according to a teaching plan. The plan outlines what the teacher will do in an attempt to foster certain learner behaviors and should reflect the desired outcomes. If the objectives are identified in behavioral terms, they can be used both as the basis for the teaching plan and later as the criteria for evaluation. An example of the objectives and a sample of the teaching plan appear in Table 8-1.

The teaching plan emanates from the staff development process and is an essential tool in committing yourself to what you have decided about the facts you have. The plan is designed to meet a learning need or a group of needs. The need, in relationship to other factors such as agency goals, leads to a formulation of a general objective for planning a particular offering. In order to have the learners meet the objectives within a realistic time period, it may be necessary to identify certain prerequisites in the plan. Prerequisites include assigning selected readings, designating certain knowledge (for example, basic anatomy of the heart), identifying certain clinical skills (for example, starting an intravenous infusion according to agency policies), or limiting the clinical practice of the learners (for example, registered nurse with one year's experience in maternal nursing). Obviously it is not necessary to have prerequisites, but if they are established, they must be made clear to the learners.

From the general objectives for the offering, the specific goals and the topics to be included are determined. These should include knowledge, skills, and attitudes appropriate to meeting the need. In formulating a teaching plan or class outline, all of the behavioral objectives should be identified as well as

Table 8-1. Teaching plan

Content	Methods and aids	Behavioral objectives
Identify main points and all major subpoints.	Designate teaching-learning methods as well as all aids to be used (alternative approach).	Place behavioral objectives in line with content for evaluation purposes.

the general flow of content and the teaching methods. Alternative approaches need to be considered and may be identified parenthetically in an outline for future reference. Additionally, it may be desirable to identify the teacher and the time block. These plans should be kept as a matter of record, so that the actual results of an offering can be compared to the projected ones.

Time schedule and staff assignment. A time schedule should be used to show each educator's class and clinical schedule. Additionally, if clinicians or outside speakers are involved in learning offerings, this should be noted on the schedule. Thus at a glance it can be determined where the staff development educators are located and what learning offerings are scheduled for the designated time. These schedules usually are made out on a monthly basis.

Although staff assignments may vary, one of the best methods is based on clinical expertise. It is not possible for all staff development educators to be experts in that field as well as in all of the clinical areas. Therefore in making assignments, the educator's area of expertise should be considered. If there is no staff development educator with a particular expertise, there may be others within the agency who have the needed knowledge and whose teaching ability could be developed. Thus the most knowledgeable person would be made available.

• • •

In designing the offering, emphasis must be placed on the experiences that will reinforce the positive behaviors that are expected in the output phase. Without this reinforcement, the expected output might not be attained.

Implementation

The actual presentation of the offering is the next step. As designated by the broken line in Fig. 1-2, climate setting again enters the picture. Climate setting refers to the creation of a comfortable learning atmosphere. If time is taken to make adults comfortable and they are allowed to get to know each other, the resultant output may be greater because each learner has used not only the educator's information but also the other people's ideas. One way to "break the ice" might be to introduce the offering and state its objectives. Once the learners have been familiarized with their purpose in attending a specific offering, they might next take time to become acquainted. If round tables accommodating six to seven persons are being used, each group could be given ten to fifteen minutes to exchange information about themselves. For example, some individuals might want others to know their career goals, whereas others may want to discuss their families. Each person might be asked to identify their individual expectations of the offering. Depending on the offering, the individuals could perhaps introduce each other to the whole group or identify something they have learned about someone in their group that had not been known before. They might be asked to identify past successes or failures related to the offering. Finally, refreshments could be served and the stage for learning set by indicating the methods to be used. Questions should be entertained as the discussion proceeds.

Once the climate has been set, it is time to implement the learning offering. The previously developed outline is the basis for implementing the offering. It has specified content, teaching methods and aids, as well as behavioral objectives. Thus it states why an offering has been implemented, how it should be carried out, and how the results might be evaluated.

Evaluation

As seen in Fig. 1-2, evaluation is a constant, ongoing process at each and every step of the development and implementation of any given effort. Although evaluation is discussed here as the end step of the process phase, this is by no means its only function. In terms of the overall effort, a reevaluation of the learners' profiles may be needed at each step. If evaluation is undertaken only after implementation, significant information may be neglected and the potential of the offering lessened.

Evaluation should also include the learners' opinions of the instruction. Their suggestions might involve changes in content, methods of instruction, or facilities. If nothing is going to be done with their comments, participants should not be asked to supply their opinions. Nothing can be more frustrating for learners than to receive a response that indicates their ideas were superfluous.

Evaluation, in addition, includes an analysis of the output. How the learner is able to use the new information indicates the success of the offering. If the environment is not conducive to using this information, the situation should be analyzed and the necessary changes made. Rather than attempting to bring about gradual change on all units, it might be wiser to effect total change on a single unit before moving on to another.

If the end product is not that which was anticipated, the input or selection of the process may not have been the most appropriate for the given situation. If success is achieved,

however, there should be apparent differences in performance. For example, several electrical hazards are found in the emergency room. A nearby university is offering a two-day seminar on electrical hazards, the offering is evaluated and the head nurse informed that it might be useful to some of the nurses. If these people attend the offering and learn from it, electrical hazards will most likely be reduced.

• • •

Nord,[1] in referring to his instructional development system, relates these three factors (input, process, and output) with the three letters A, E, and T. Assembled in different ways, these three letters can produce the words "ate," "eat," and "tea," each having a different meaning. Similarly, the way in which input, process, and output are related can produce different effects.

Medearis and Popiel[2] adapted a model to demonstrate the never-ending training cycle. The parts are identified as (1) determine and validate needs, (2) set goals and define specific objectives, (3) plan course and design learning activities, (4) implement plan, (5) select and prepare resources, (6) evaluate using objectives as criteria, and (7) recycle the process.

If only one point could be made about the interrelation of the three factors, it should be the necessity of evaluating the output in reconsidering the input and process. Without such feedback it may never be known why changes did not occur.

DESIGNING COMPONENTS

No matter what the staff development process is called, it contains certain core elements such as an introduction to a new position and new information necessary for professional development. These elements must be considered in the organization of the program. In 1958 Miller wrote one of the first manuals on in-service education, and for many years her National League for Nursing publication has been referred to as the "bible of in-service education." She divided in-service education into four areas of personnel needs:

1. A need for an introduction to their job.
2. A need for training in both the manual and behavioral skills associated with their jobs.
3. A need for development of leadership and management abilities.
4. A need for continuing investigation of the real potentialities of their jobs.°

These needs were designated as orientation, skill training, leadership and management development, and continuing education.

Later, Stopera and Scully[3] suggested another way of organizing learning activities. They identified specific curriculum content that was self-sustaining, rather than totally dependent on leadership. They proposed five major categories in their structure:

1.0 Orientation
  1.1 General
  1.2 Unit orientation
2.0 Technical/professional training programs
3.0 Leadership/management training programs
  3.1 Leadership training
  3.2 Management programs
4.0 Safety training programs
5.0 Continuing education
  5.1 Hospital-wide programs
  5.2 Out-of-house programs
  5.3 Other training programs

Thus Stopera and Scully have used Miller's approach but have identified safety as a separate entity and have expanded continuing education to include out-of-house programs.

A third way of organizing learning offerings is to distinguish two major components, orientation and continuing education. Essential to this approach is the incorporation of skill training and leadership development as integral parts in each component. This is an adaptation of Miller's approach.

°Miller, M. A.: Inservice education for hospital nursing personnel, New York, 1958, National League for Nursing.

Orientation

Orientation is the process whereby a new staff member is introduced to a particular work setting. The orientation program should be conducted prior to new employees assuming responsibility for the positions for which they were hired. This definition implies that individual needs are recognized whether the person is new to the agency or new to a particular position within the agency.

When planning orientation for a group of learners, the role expectations must be identified. Position descriptions can be used and the staff development educator should have a knowledge of them. Skills inventory and preservice profiles also will aid the educator when planning orientation. It may be necessary to make some generalizations about the learners before a profile is developed. Generally a profile is not developed before the learner is employed. Therefore some generalizations might be made about "new graduates," "graduates from associate degree programs," or "graduates from this particular school" in order to develop a basic outline. The orientation may be modified depending on the individual learners. For example, a nurse with a great deal of practical experience may need little clinical assistance. However, a new graduate may have difficulty attending the classes because of extensive clinical instruction and the need to do additional reading. Perhaps she requires an extended orientation period to meet the defined expectations.

Although different agencies use various approaches to the organization and content of orientation, it is assumed that there is certain basic knowledge needed by employees before they can function within designated positions. This knowledge is considered a basic core element.

There is certain information that all employees must have regardless of such factors as classification, educational preparation, experiential background, and role expectations. Depending on the setting, this content could be limited or expanded, but it generally includes information about the agency, the health care philosophy, fire and safety programs, and personnel policies. Many agencies also include a tour to acquaint all employees with the physical facility. If it is really crucial that certain employees (for instance, maintenance personnel) know more about the physical plant, additional guidance should be planned. Frequently this session is conducted by the personnel department or the training department of the agency.

Other content is geared to a specific group or even to an individual. This additional information may relate to a group on the basis of various differentiations such as (1) classification—registered nurses or licensed practical nurses; (2) clinical area—psychiatric nursing or maternal nursing; (3) educational preparation—master's graduate or associate degree graduate; (4) role expectations—staff nurse or nurse clinician; and (5) experiential background—a new graduate or a registered nurse with several years' experience in a specific clinical area.

It is beneficial to all concerned to have the objectives and class schedules in a written format (see Appendix, Exhibits G and H). How content is organized within the overall effort of orientation depends on a variety of factors within a given agency, and it would be wise to consider the following variables:

1. Size of agency
2. Philosophy of agency, nursing practice, and staff development
3. Instructional staff
4. Resources available
5. Staff development policies
6. Staffing patterns

The number and types of new employees at any given time can dictate the organization. Additionally, a wide variance of needs among the employees can create difficulties for the staff development educator.

The philosophies of the agency concerning nursing practice and staff development can influence how content is organized. If the setting is highly centralized and there is little variance among the clinical services and role

expectations, a great deal of content can be presented uniformly. If, however, the agency organization is decentralized, the new employees must be involved within their respective specialities as soon and as much as possible.

One of the most critical factors to assess is the instructional staff. If there are few staff development educators and the frequency of hiring is not controlled, there may be difficulty in organizing instruction. If such a situation exists, it generally is possible to organize the content with regard to individual needs. Additionally, head nurses and supervisors might be utilized in teaching, providing this function is a part of their role expectations.

The various resources within and outside the agency should be considered also. The personnel director might discuss personnel policies. A safety officer or the chairman of the safety committee could discuss and demonstrate appropriate safety precautions. Someone from a local college, university, or professional or community organization may provide some portion of the orientation content. For example, a local heart association might offer a cardiopulmonary resuscitation course that could be incorporated into the basic orientation. If, however, these resources do not exist, the people seem unable to make effective points, or they cannot participate on a regular basis, the staff development educators may have to meet the learners' needs by themselves.

Although many agencies have not defined their staff development policies in writing, the policies do exist. For example, many agencies have a policy (whether written or implied) relating to the time interval for hiring new employees. If the agency hires new nursing personnel every two weeks or once a month, the organization of the content would be considerably different than if the hiring took place once a week or whenever someone appeared on the doorstep. Obviously it is desirable to have a policy that allows for planned, organized efforts.

Finally, a factor that most of us are familiar with is staffing. At those times when there is a real need for additional help, everyone wants new employees "now!" The pressure to "get the people on the unit" frequently influences how rapidly staff development educators incorporate clinical practice in the orientation effort. Limited staffing may affect the organization of orientation in another way, too. It may be difficult to expect assistance from the staff if they are already reduced in numbers, if the patient census is abnormally high, or if the patient care requirements are greater than normal. While this factor needs to be considered, it certainly should not determine how the content is organized.

Having analyzed these six factors—size of agency, philosophy of agency regarding nursing practice and staff development, instructional staff, resources available, staff development policies, and staffing patterns—it can then be decided what content should be

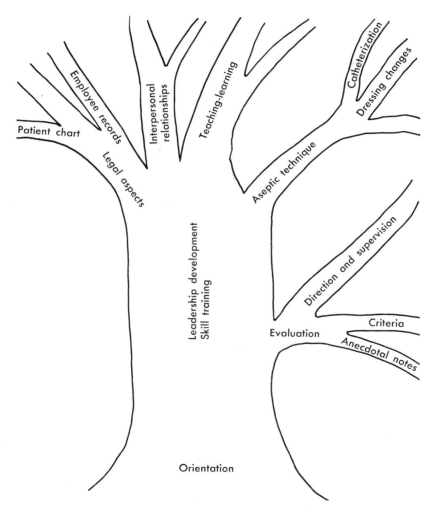

Fig. 8-1. Centralized-decentralized orientation. Basic knowledge and skills in orientation can be centralized and decentralized. The foundations are made centrally and the specifics can branch into various decentralized areas.

centralized and what should be decentralized. Information that is needed by all of the employees can be offered on a centralized basis. However, content relating to specific areas of practice should be implemented and evaluated in a decentralized manner. An example of material to be presented through a combined approach would be records and reports. The centralized core content would be depicted by the basic chart used throughout the agency. If a few of the learners were assigned to maternity nursing, they would meet their orientation needs by gaining specific knowledge about birth and delivery records on a decentralized basis. An example of how such content can be core and branched is given in Fig. 8-1.

Another example of a centralized-decentralized approach is patient assessment. The core content, the basic principles of assessing patient needs, would be given on a centralized basis, but the branch content—implementation and evaluation—would be decentralized. One of the staff development educators or the head nurse could provide specific clinical content to new employees on an individualized or small-group basis. If, however, the situation does not permit this approach, it would be necessary to incorporate specialized or selectively relevant content centrally. One must be alert to potential boredom, however, on the part of learners to whom some information does not apply. One must also be alert to a different output than that expected when there are "distracting" factors such as much specialized content in a general discussion. Another approach to incorporating specialized content centrally is through scheduling. For example, from the total group of nurses, there may be two who need knowledge about traction equipment. When this subject is discussed, only the two who need the information will be involved, the others might participate in a self-learning activity or remain in the clinical area.

Throughout this planning phase, it must be remembered that the objectives of orientation are the primary consideration. The identifica-

tion of the skills of new employees provides a data base for comparison with the objectives of orientation. The discrepancies are the learners' needs. One of the best approaches is to examine the position descriptions and organize the role expectations around central themes. For example, some appropriate divisions for a staff nurse position description might be nursing care, interpersonal relationships, teaching-learning, and direction and supervision. The knowledge needed in these aspects should be centralized. The subsequent evaluation of how this learning is being applied in the clinical areas would occur throughout the orientation period.

An example of such an approach is seen in Fig. 8-1. As seen in this figure, skill training and leadership development are integral parts of orientation. One of the most common examples of skill training within orientation is that of nurse assistant programs. The basic training course is the most familiar method of skill training. Although these programs vary among agencies, the majority include routine skills that do not involve in-depth clinical judgment but are needed by the consumers of the service. These skills usually include making beds, giving baths, feeding patients, providing back care, performing some routine procedures, recording certain kinds of information, collecting specimens, and cleaning equipment (see Appendix, Exhibit I). Although it is assumed that other personnel have learned these skills in their preservice programs, it is necessary to observe them in the clinical areas to be certain that the skills are present.

Different groups of employees may have different skill needs. For example, nurse assistants may need body mechanics skills (see Appendix, Exhibit J), while registered nurses may need interaction skills. As seen in the above example, the term "skills" denotes more than just manual proficiency. The ability to conduct an interview may require as much practice as making an occupied bed. Clinical experience or simulated experience is important in both examples.

Leadership development is another integral part of orientation. Stodgill's definition of leadership as "... the process of influencing the activities of an organized group in its efforts toward goal setting and goal achievement,"[4] is acceptable for our purposes. According to this definition, there are many leaders within a given clinical setting. In an orientation effort, leadership may focus on the team leader's role in holding team members accountable, in evaluating team members, or in leading group discussion. Whatever is included should be clearly delineated for the learners (see Appendix, Exhibit K). The content covered in this aspect of orientation depends on the role expectations of the various exployees within the agency. It would be difficult to adopt another agency's program if the position descriptions, learners, organizational structure, and philosophy were not the same. The only way of knowing if the right program has been offered is through an analysis of output.

In summary, there are some specific content areas that need to be included in any orientation. The following list may prove a useful guide.

1. Introductions
2. History of agency and patient population
3. Philosophy and objectives of agency and department
4. Organization plan—agency, department, nursing unit
5. Role expectations
6. Nursing care standards
7. Policies
8. Safety
9. Disaster and emergency preparedness
10. Physical facilities—nursing care areas, other departments, library
11. Records and reports
12. Staff development offerings
13. Procedures
14. Legal and ethical responsibilities
15. Evaluation

In reviewing the staff development process (Fig. 1-2), consideration should be given to the employees' role expectations, needed modifications based on individual data, and what is most essential to the function of the agency. What best meets the agency's needs at the present time must be determined.

Whatever the organization of content and experiences, it should be remembered that orientation can be centralized as well as decentralized, and that it prepares an employee to function within defined role expectations. The success of the orientation program is measured in the output stage.

Continuing education

Continuing education is that part of staff development designed to assist nursing personnel to gain new knowledge and skills, review and add to knowledge already gained, investigate new approaches in nursing, and strengthen their clinical competencies. Continuing education should foster innovative and creative approaches to the nursing care of patients for the purpose of achieving more effective behavior in nursing practice that improves the quality of patient care and thus increases job satisfaction.

For many years the improvement of nursing knowledge and skills has been promoted. The American Nurses' Association has developed standards for nursing service and nursing education, and state boards of nursing have been involved with the implementation of standards. Health care agencies have supported continuing education, but only recently have there been many efforts in planning and implementation.

Today all health care agencies have the responsibility of affording their employees opportunities to continue their education and to develop themselves as members of the health care team. Most departments within health care agencies offer some type of continuing education. It is not uncommon to see program notices for dietary, housekeeping, physical therapy, and other departments. Nursing, however, was the forerunner in offering continuing education within staff development. Today many members of the nursing profession participate in programs offered by the agency as well as those outside the agency in order to broaden their knowledge and skills.

In continuing education, as in orientation, there is certain core knowledge that all employees must have regardless of such factors as classification, educational preparation, experiential background, and role expectations. For example, safety is a critical factor, and knowledge related to it is essential for all personnel. In orientation all aspects of patient and personnel safety are introduced and discussed in order to promote a safe environment for all concerned. For instance, personnel must know the correct procedure for evacuating patients. And if there is a structural change in the facility that makes a new and more effective method of evacuation possible, continuing education offerings should be conducted so that the personnel may become acquainted with it. This type of content is considered continuing education because new knowledge is being presented; orientation, on the other hand, involves basic knowledge that the personnel need in order to function in their roles.

Other continuing education offerings may be geared to a group or even to an individual. As with orientation, the content may relate to a group on the basis of various differentiations such as (1) classification—registered nurses or licensed practical nurses; (2) clinical areas—coronary care nursing or surgical nursing; (3) role expectations—staff nurse or nurse clinician; (4) educational preparation—master's graduate or associate degree graduate; and (5) experiential background—a new graduate or a registered nurse with several years' experience in a specific clinical area.

How this continuing education content is organized depends on those variables that were outlined and discussed under orientation—size of an agency; philosophy of the agency, nursing practice, and staff development; instructional staff; resources available; staff development policies; and staffing patterns.

The size of the agency may affect the organization of continuing education offerings. For example, in a large agency a certain offering might be presented forty-five times in order to have all the personnel attend, while in a smaller agency, six offerings may suffice. Therefore a larger agency is likely to employ more audiovisual aids because of the repetition of offerings.

The philosophy of the agency, nursing practice, and staff development influence the continuing education program. If there is extreme centralization, the educator will find it difficult to meet the needs of all personnel. For example, one of the role expectations for a staff nurse might be the ability to function as a charge nurse on a given shift. While common learning experiences can be offered centrally, it is virtually impossible to prepare each staff nurse for a charge position on a specific service on such a basis. Decentralization, however, takes into account the differences between each unit and its patient population.

The number of educators needed for an effective continuing education program is always difficult to assess. The size of the agency, philosophy, budget, role expectations of personnel, as well as the kind of continuing education offerings will influence this decision. However, there are certain questions that can be asked in reaching a decision.

1. Am I expected to reach employees on all shifts?
2. What support systems are available that could help in teaching?
3. How do I as the staff development educator function in my job? What role do I assume? Am I a facilitator? How many nonteaching functions do I have?
4. Am I using educational technology systems personnel for assistance in teaching?
5. Am I reaching people at the most opportune moment?
6. How centralized or decentralized are we in our organization?
7. What are the needs for continuing education?

After these questions have been answered, it should be easier to assess needs and to determine the number of educators needed for effective continuing education.

Depending on the learning resources within the agency, the use of outside resources may or may not be necessary. When organizing the continuing education offerings, the first step should be a determination of resources within the agency. It may be found that there are health care personnel who are adept at teaching and very willing to share their knowledge. Also, there may be other agencies in the community that would like to share services. For example, one agency might do all the coronary care teaching; a second agency, all the nurse assistants training; and a third agency, the instruction on geriatric nursing. Such cooperation may or may not be written into a contractual agreement. The sharing of hardware or software is also common among smaller hospitals. In fact, with the cost factor today, larger hospitals are beginning to share software, too. "Trade-offs" are also in effect between some agencies; "If you send students to my agency for instruction, I'll use yours for a continuing education effort." This "trade-off" technique could be particularly useful to an agency having students affiliated with it and will likely be used more in the future.

Staff development policies, either written or implied, will make a difference in the organization of continuing education. For example, if there is a policy that makes attendance at continuing education offerings mandatory, the sessions must be scheduled so that all of the various shifts may attend. Thus such a policy greatly affects the organization of continuing education.

Staffing patterns always play an important part in continuing education. The scheduling of a given offering must be given careful consideration. In hospitals as well as other agencies there are always certain days of the week on which the greatest number of nursing personnel within a specific area are available. It may be advisable to schedule the same offering several times during the week. For example, an offering is being held for head nurses, and in order to make it available to all of them, it must be scheduled two times a week.

The six factors just discussed are all interrelated in the planning of continuing education. They cannot be separated when planning leadership development, advanced interviewing skills, or patient assessment offerings. The way in which the offerings are organized will be dependent on these factors.

Emphasis must be placed on providing opportunities for learning new knowledge, skills, and attitudes if the learners are to approach self-actualization. The role of the nurse is gradually changing from that of data collector to data interpreter. The "subservient" role the nurse once played is changing to an interdependent relationship with the other members of the health team. In this new role, nurses are better able to meet organizational and consumer goals. This change is essential to the improvement of nursing practice and to career satisfaction as well as to better patient care.

Inherent in the process of employees' developing their potentials are the concepts of reward and reinforcement. While many people enjoy participating in continuing education offerings, they may become frustrated if their efforts are not recognized. If an agency views continuing education as a part of an individual's development, it must be clearly defined as a role expectation and must be considered in evaluation. If, for example, several offerings were designated as "mandatory" and one of the nurses did not attend any of them, this should be considered in evaluating that employee. Similarly, if another employee has attended all "mandatory" offerings plus several additional ones and demonstrates the expected performance behaviors, then this, too, should be considered. If expectations of continuing education efforts are not reinforced clinically, the employees may not see any value in continuing their education. It is important, therefore, that the educational record be reviewed prior to writing an evaluation of an employee, and that the employee knows such a review will take place.

The negative aspect of reward and reinforcement is punishment. It, too, can influence personnel. Some agencies reduce benefits or wages if employees do not attend mandatory offerings, while others issue written warnings. Although this system is not so effective as its positive counterpart, it does control behavior. There is a danger with this approach that although the personnel are forced to attend class, they still may not change their behavior in the clinical area. Therefore, before negative reinforcement is made, consideration should be given to other methods of holding them accountable.

The selection of mandatory offerings must be made carefully. Generally attendance should be required at offerings related to a major change in a safety measure, thereby showing that all employees were informed of the proposed change prior to its initiation. Obviously it is essential for staff development educators to schedule mandatory offerings so that all personnel may attend during their working shifts. This may be difficult in agencies that have a significant percentage of their staff working on a part-time basis, especially if some members work only one or two days a week. Hence it may be necessary to institute a self-instruction program for certain members of the staff and then carefully evaluate their related performance.

Other offerings that may be mandatory might involve legal aspects (for example, a change in the charting procedure) or the approach to nursing care (for example, moving from a functional approach to the team or primary approach). It must be remembered that if all offerings are made mandatory and there is not a system of reward and reinforcement or punishment, a situation may arise analogous to that of the little boy who cried "wolf"—the employees will never know what is truly significant.

When certain offerings have been designated as essential to continuing education, they should be incorporated in the yearly and monthly schedules. The monthly schedule may reflect all learning offerings (centralized and decentralized); or there may be two schedules—one for all centralized offerings and another for all decentralized offerings. It is also possible to prepare two monthly schedules, with regard to orientation and continuing education. Exhibits L and M in the Appendix are examples of a yearly and monthly schedule.

Depending on the number of employees, it may be advisable to limit registration for the offerings. In such an event it would be necessary to devise some method by which to identify the learners, what they view as their learning needs, and what their past educational experiences include (basic and continuing). This information can be used to modify certain content and approaches or to redefine the purpose of a particular offering.

As in orientation, skill training and leadership development are interwoven aspects of continuing education. Within this context, however, the skills are new and build on those previously learned. Depending on individual background, the learning of a particular skill may be classified as orientation for one, but continuing education for another. While it is not necessary to make a major distinction between orientation and continuing education, the difference between the two must be taken into account in evaluating output. If the information is given as a review, the individual would be expected to exhibit changed behavior more rapidly than if the content were new.

If a skill is presented in continuing education that the nurses have not encountered before, in-depth content must be prepared in order to facilitate understanding. Whether the skill is manual or intellectual, practice sessions should be incorporated so that the learners can develop their new skills. These sessions may be a part of the structured class, or they may be decentralized and involve specific individuals within the clinical setting. Whatever the case, proper guidance is most important in this phase.

Continuing education efforts in leadership development attempt to develop the learner's abilities to work with people. Some offerings may be promotional (see Appendix, Exhibit N), designed to groom certain individuals for advancement to positions with added authority and responsibility. Depending on the agency's needs, certain basic leadership content might be offered at designated times throughout the year so that all persons needing this educational experience could avail themselves of it.

In many agencies, promotion can occur without a concurrent change in job classification. For example, nurse assistants are often designated as being of group I or II, with the latter assuming additional responsibilities. Also, many agencies categorize their licensed practical nurses on the basis of whether or not they have had a medication course. Further differentiation may be made with regard to the level of competency exhibited in the fulfillment of role expectations. Some agencies also distinguish between the clinical and administrative abilities of their registered nurses. Some of these advanced positions are achieved as a result of demonstrated performance behaviors that qualified the individuals for participation in the agency's program for the advanced classification. A portion of a promotional offering for nurse assistants appears in Exhibit O of the Appendix.

Whether an offering is promotional, mandatory, or neither, certain guidelines should be followed in its implementation. The offering must be consistent with the objectives of the agency and the philosophy regarding nursing practice and staff development. An interdisciplinary approach may be used in its planning as well as implementation.° The budget for a given offering, if one is required, includes planning, implementing, and evaluating expenses. Inherent in the offering are the concepts of adult learning. Various needs are identified that may require particular teaching methods and aids. Behavioral objectives are designated for each offering and are used for evaluation. Evaluation is made in terms of performance behaviors (output). How the offerings are designed and implemented varies from agency to agency; there

°Many offerings currently are available to various disciplines but are planned by one.

is no general format that is applicable in every case. However, it can be said unequivocally that the output will depend largely on how the needs are met.

REFERENCES

1. Nord, J. R.: A search for meaning, Audiovis. Instr. **16**:11, Dec., 1971.
2. Medearis, N. D., and Popiel, E. S.: Guidelines for organizing inservice education, J. Nurs. Admin. **1**(4): 30, 1971.
3. Stopera, V., and Scully, D.: A workable organizational model for staff development departments, J. Cont. Educ. Nurs. **3**(6):14, 1972.
4. Stodgill, R. M.: Leadership, membership and organization, Psychol. Bull. **47**:4, Jan., 1950.

BIBLIOGRAPHY

American Nurses' Association: An interim statement on continuing education in nursing, Kansas City, Mo., 1972, The Association.
Cantor. M.: Education for quality care, J. Nurs. Admin. **3**(1):49, 1973.
Cantor, N.: The teaching-learning process, New York, 1953, Dryden Press.
Cooper, S. S., and Hornback, M. I.: Continuing nursing education, New York, 1973, McGraw-Hill Book Co.
Del Bueno, D. J.: Verifying the nurse's knowledge of pharmacology, Nurs. Outlook **20**:462, 1972.
Heffernan, B. M.: Keeping nurses up to date, Nurs. Outlook **20**:265, 1972.
Holloman, C. R.: Leadership and headship: there is a difference, Personnel Admin. **31**:38, July-Aug. 1968.
Houle, C. O.: The design of education, San Francisco, 1972, Jossey-Bass Inc., Publishers.
Knowles, M.: The modern practice of adult education, New York, 1970, Association Press.
Lysaught, J. P.: Continuing education: necessity and opportunity, J. Cont. Educ. Nurs. **1**(5):5, 1970.
McGregor, D.: The human side of enterprise, New York, 1960, McGraw-Hill Book Co.
Mager, R. F.: Developing attitudes toward learning, Palo Alto, Calif., 1968, Fearon Publishers.
Miller, M. A.: Inservice education for hospital nursing personnel, New York, 1958, National League for Nursing.
Swansburg, R. C.: Inservice education, New York, 1968, G. P. Putnam's Sons.
Tyler, R. W.: Basic principles of curriculum and instruction, Chicago, 1949, University of Chicago Press.
Waller, M., and Davids, D.: Performance profiles based on nursing activity records, J. Nurs. Admin. **2**(5):61, 1972.
Western Interstate Commission for Higher Education: Continuing education in nursing, Boulder, Colo., 1969, The Commission.
Yoder, P. S.: Planning for learning through the professional association, J. Cont. Educ. Nurs. **3**(5):22, 1972.

9

Selecting teaching methods and aids

DOROTHY H. COYE

This may sound like the repetitious beating of an old and very tired horse, but the simple fact seems to be that continuing education, like continuing education years ago, is obsessed with the idea that exposure to the learned assures learning. Yet each generation rediscovers the fact that in the end it is the learner who must do the learning, and no amount of communication by lecture, by book, by film, by radio or by television will make the slightest difference unless he does something with what he receives.°

The selection of an effective and economical teaching method or aid to assist learners to do something with what they learn is a provocative and exciting challenge encountered by today's concerned staff development educator: challenging, since the steady acquisition of new knowledge in the field of teaching and learning provides an increasing number of instructional approaches from which to choose; challenging, too, since the impermanence of all knowledge requires periodic reorganization of educational programs if the learning needs of those who must maintain their skills are to be met; provoking, when the teaching method selected fails to produce changes in behavior; and exciting, when a new approach yields an interested learner who indeed "does something with what he receives."

Teaching methods are simply ways to provide learning experiences. Methods vary somewhat according to whether the learners must (1) receive information, (2) be shown objects or procedures, or (3) participate ac-

tively in their own learning. Most teaching approaches involve content and relevant materials. No method is all "right" or all "wrong." The staff development educator selects a method that best facilitates the learning experience, giving consideration to the economy of time, materials, and energy as well. Teaching aids may enhance a method, but they are not methods in and of themselves—they may help or hinder the transfer of content, depending on the skill with which the staff development educator uses them.

Many references to single-task orientation are made in this chapter. Emphasis is placed on the concept that the whole job is only the sum of its separate tasks. Each task, whether simple or complex, utilizing manual or intellectual skills, is performed separately, can be classified, and therefore can be taught separately. It is emphasized further that orientation to the whole job is accomplished by learning the individual tasks.

In this chapter some of the considerations involved in the selection of instructional methods and aids for a staff development program will be presented.

°Miller, G. E.: The continuing education of physicians, N. Engl. J. Med. **269:**298, 1963.

PHILOSOPHY AND SELECTION

The beliefs about staff development, identified and expressed by the staff development educator in a statement of philosophy, provide a functional basis for the selection of teaching methods.[1] If, for example, the philosophy of staff development reflects a belief that relevancy to the work should guide the teaching program, that learning needs are best identified and provided for in the area where the work is performed, and further that the involvement of the staff in its own learning is desirable, then a decentralized teaching program would be applied. In this approach, employees are assisted in identifying their own learning needs on the unit and actively participate in meeting them. To implement this philosophy, the staff development educator provides centralized continuing education courses designed to assist key members of the nursing staff to improve their skills in directing and teaching other staff members as well as patients and their families. The staff development educator thus becomes a teaching consultant to the unit staff by offering assistance in the selection and utilization of teaching methods.

When the statement of belief is used as a basis for selection, useful goals, objectives, and teaching approaches are easier to identify. Justification of the program becomes difficult when the approaches selected are in conflict with the stated philosophy.

ECONOMICS AND SELECTION

The economics involved in the use of teaching methods is an essential consideration. Low budgets and high costs in all areas of education are a common problem today. Education for health care personnel is usually subsidized by the consumers of the service who demand and deserve a return on their investment. The staff development educator has an obligation to waste neither the dollar outlay of the health care consumers nor the time of the learners through poor selection of teaching methods. Time is one of the most expensive items in the budget. While the cost of preparing a self-instructional teaching unit may seem high when compared to that of preparing a lecture, it is actually less expensive if the lecture does not improve the quality of patient care either because of poor preparation, organization, or delivery. Even when a lecture is well prepared and delivered, the learning that occurs may be limited. A self-instructional package, though time-consuming and involving costs for supplies and materials, may produce a higher learning yield and thus be the most economical method.[2] This choice should be influenced by the extent and complexity of the desired learning. It would be extravagant to prepare a programmed instruction lesson concerning the location of unit supplies. However, it would be economical to prepare a programmed instruction lesson on fire prevention. Costs involved in any selected teaching approach for staff development may be difficult to justify. The teacher may select an appropriate and economical method and use it well; the audiovisual material may be of high quality, accurate, and relevant to the learning needs; and the learner may learn. Yet, as Cantor[3] points out, the learner may choose not to translate newly acquired skills, knowledge, and understanding into practice. Many variables influence human behavior and education is but one of them. Nor is it easy to defend the selected method if patient care is unaffected. Thus the source of funding must be considered in the selection of the teaching method.

ORIENTATION AND SELECTION

Orientation is the process of introducing an employee to a new position and to new tasks. The selection of instructional methods for orientation programs is concerned essentially with teaching tasks. Bernotavicz and Wallington[4] suggest an approach for developing a curriculum to orient employees to their assigned positions and to their new tasks. This study, designed to provide data to restructure selected jobs and to develop training approaches for these jobs, revealed that (1) any job is comprised of separate tasks, each with definite starting and stopping points; (2) what *gets done* and what you *do* are not the same; that is, what you *do* is a series of separate tasks, the results of which are the whole of what *gets done;* and (3) all tasks involve working with either data, people, or things, and orientation to each task usually deals with only one area at a time. For example, the nurse assistant who organizes the day's patient assignment, the nurse who withholds digitalis when the patient's pulse rate is low, and the nurse who assesses the patient's needs through observation are all performing tasks that involve working with information. Each of these tasks can be classified, has an identifiable beginning and end, and can be taught singly. To illustrate further, the head nurse who requests the nursing staff to develop a new approach to a procedure; the nurse assistant who is engaged in conversation with a disoriented geriatric patient; or the emergency room nurse who must inform parents of the death of their teen-aged son due to drug overdose are all performing tasks that involve working with people. Each task has an identifiable start and finish and can be taught as a single segment. Tasks that involve working with things are not difficult to imagine and need not be illustrated here.

An application of Bernotavicz and Wallington's concept in the selection of teaching methods for orientation is used in the following example. Consider that one of the nurse's jobs is to "start I.V.'s." According to Bernotavicz and Wallington, this job would be comprised of several tasks, each with a definite beginning and end and that could be classified as involving either data, people, or things. Since each of these three areas requires a different instructional approach, the selection of a method to teach the nurse how to "start I.V.'s" first involves classification of the tasks involved. Does it involve learning *data?* Most institutions limit the type of intravenous solutions the nurse is permitted to administer. Thus one task involves working with a list of information. Can class time be devoted to the memorization of lists? Can this information

be printed on inexpensive duplicator paper in a small pocket-sized handout that briefly highlights the information to be learned, reduces class time, and provides a quick and available reference as well (Fig. 9-1)? Can the list be posted in a prominent and conveniently located place for quick reference? In all probability the cost of the printed handout is less than the cost of the learner's classroom time. In any case, the nurse will learn the information through actual practice.

It must next be determined whether or not the task involves *working with people.* Of course, instructions to the patient about the intravenous therapy are required as part of the procedure. Learning this task, however, is not a major objective in teaching the nurse how to "start I.V.'s" and would be included only as a brief review of previously learned information. Finally, it is established that the tasks to be learned are involved with *things—* I.V. containers, tubing, needles, veins, flow regulation valves, and records. The selected teaching method is, of course, demonstration and supervised practice.

This teaching method selection may be illustrated by another example. If, because of a revision in policy, the nurse now will be giving U 100 insulin instead of the traditional types (U 40 and U 80), some orientation to the revised policy is in order. The nurse already knows how to measure insulin in units, how to inject insulin, and how to approach patients receiving it. Thus in this example the task to be learned involves new information. A short lecture or discussion on the differences between traditional insulin and U 100 insulin is probably the most expedient teaching method. Visual aids for the lecture should include U 100 containers and syringes as well as a brief handout containing the basic information to be used for later reference. The handout is important when the lecture method is used since retention of information received through this teaching method is often limited and short-lived. However, the printed materials in this example are supplemental and should not be used in place of class attendance.

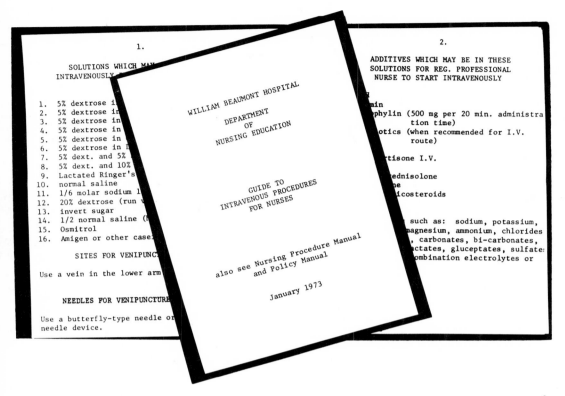

Fig. 9-1. Pocket-sized handout briefly highlights information to be learned, reduces class time, and provides a quick reference. (Courtesy William Beaumont Hospital, Royal Oak, Mich.)

Selection of teaching methods for task orientation involves several considerations. The number, availability, and classifications of learners, complexity of tasks to be learned, and facilities and materials required are a few of these considerations. One problem that staff development educators face with some regularity is the selection of an instructional approach when a new task involves either the entire nursing staff or all employees in one category (Fig. 9-2). Television has helped to solve this problem at William Beaumont Hospital. However, forty-eight closed-circuit TV classes are required to reach all nursing employees. All unit conference rooms are equipped with TV monitors. The schedule of forty-eight classes, which begins at the end of one week and continues through the weekend and into the first part of the following week,

allows for days off, part- and full-time schedules, and the various shift assignments. In addition, scheduling several classes for each shift on successive days provides for small groups of learners, avoids depletion of the unit staff at any one time, and reduces overtime costs by providing a sufficient number of classes during scheduled working hours. When the content to be learned is needed by all nursing employees and is such that personal face-to-face instruction is required, the schedule is usually doubled. It also means that the instruction must be shared by all staff development educators, head nurses, and supervisors. When the same content is taught by several people, there is a danger that the material may be expanded, reduced, or misinterpreted. When multiple lectures or demonstrations are required in order to reach many employees, it is

WILLIAM BEAUMONT HOSPITAL
Department of Nursing Education

CLASS SCHEDULE - I.V. PROCEDURE
CCTV TO ALL CONFERENCE ROOMS

| | Mon.
Jan. 12 | Mon.
Jan. 15-22 | Tues.
Jan. 16-23 | Wed.
Jan. 17-24 | Thurs.
Jan. 18-25 | Fri.
Jan. 19-26 | Sat.
Jan. 20 | Sun.
Jan. 21 |
|---|---|---|---|---|---|---|---|---|
| | | | 4:00 AM | 4:00 AM | 4:00 AM | 4:00 AM | 4:00 AM | 4:00 AM |
| | | | 4:30 AM | 4:30 AM | 4:30 AM | 4:30 AM | 4:30 AM | 4:30 AM |
| | 1:00 PM | 1:00 PM | 1:00 PM | 1:00 PM | 1:00 PM | 1:00 PM | 1:00 PM | 1:00 PM |
| | 1:30 PM | 1:30 PM | 1:30 PM | 1:30 PM | 1:30 PM | 1:30 PM | 1:30 PM | 1:30 PM |
| | 2:00 PM | 2:00 PM | 2:00 PM | 2:00 PM | 2:00 PM | 2:00 PM | | |
| | | 7:30 PM | 7:30 PM | 7:30 PM | 7:30 PM | 7:30 PM | 7:30 PM | 7:30 PM |
| | | 8:00 PM | 8:00 PM | 8:00 PM | 8:00 PM | 8:00 PM | 8:00 PM | 8:00 PM |

Personnel Approved to Supervise I.V. Practice:

Nursing Education Instructors

Clinical Nursing Coordinators

Clinical Nursing Supervisors

Assistants to Director of Clinical Nursing - PM's, Nights

Robert England, R.Ph., Pharmacy

RN's formerly assigned to I.V. Team

S. Allen and J. Oswald, Emergency Room

G. Kruckeberg and M. Slatkin, 9th Floor

RN's assigned to ICU, CCU, Kidney Unit, and Ped.

Fig. 9-2. Master class schedule designed to provide required classes for all staff during on-duty time. (Courtesy William Beaumont Hospital, Royal Oak, Mich.)

recommended that the instruction be recorded in some fashion for consistency, economy, accuracy, and validity of output. Videotapes, slides, slide-sound presentations, or programmed instruction are a few teaching aids that will help to control the content and avoid the hazards mentioned previously. Also, when information is recorded, it is available for the orientation of new employees at some later date.

SELECTION OF TEACHING METHODS FOR ORIENTATION

Most teaching methods can be adapted for use in job or task orientation. Of course, some approaches are more suitable than others. The appropriateness and limitations of several methods will be described here.

Lecture

The lecture is probably the most widely used method. It is most suitable for orienta-

tion to tasks requiring the acquisition of data or information. Many adults were taught by this method and find it a more comfortable approach than one requiring their active participation. On the other hand, most of us are not auditory learners and are easily distracted from the lecture. A pencil is dropped, a door opened, someone coughs or sneezes and the lecture point is lost. For these reasons it is important to add visual aids to the lecture. One simple aid is a printed topic outline of the lecture that provides a convenient record of the lecturer's points. The use of transparencies, slides, flip charts, or a blackboard adds visual cues that help make a lecture more meaningful. Most important of all, verbal illustrations and examples are imaginary visual aids and should be included as often as possible. Length is another important factor involved in the success of a lecture designed to orient employees to tasks. An enormously talented lecturer-instructor may be capable of holding

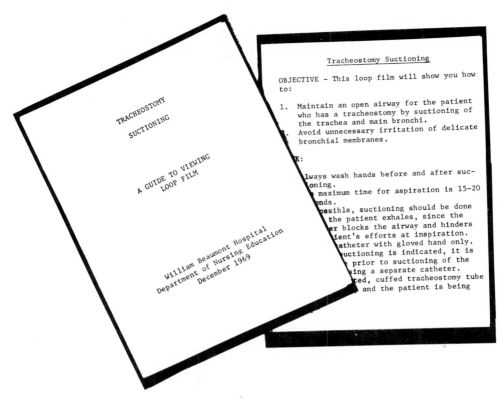

Fig. 9-3. Individual printed guides to viewing loop films make it possible to study points prior to viewing and serve as a quick reference later. (Courtesy William Beaumont Hospital, Royal Oak, Mich.)

the employees' attention throughout a forty-minute lecture. Most of us are not endowed with this talent and need to consider breaking our lectures into fifteen- or twenty-minute segments and utilizing as many visual aids as possible. The lecture method is most advantageous when used for orientation to tasks involving data, where student participation is not important. Other methods are more useful when the instruction focuses on people or things and can be facilitated by discussion or physical participation.

Demonstration

The demonstration method is best suited for teaching those tasks involved with "things." This method has the advantage of providing the instructor with instant eval-uation, since all the learners should be allowed to see, feel, and operate the equipment. Class size for adequate demonstration is necessarily limited to no more than twenty. Remember this is an orientation to tasks involving things the staff must learn to operate. A demonstration of equipment to a large audience usually falls into the category of exposure to data or information, since no opportunity to practice is provided.

Demonstration equipment should be tested and in working order before class. Audience arrangement should be such that all can see, hear, and be available to practice with the equipment or materials. It is also recommended that brief, pocket-sized handouts be designed to describe the equipment and its operation, particularly if the equipment is new and strange (Fig. 9-3). For example, the tracheostomy suctioning procedure is often an anxiety-provoking experience not only for staff members who care for patients with tracheostomies but also for family members who must care for the patients after their discharge. Since learning is more difficult when anxiety is high, a handout summarizing the procedure and supplementing the demonstration would probably be helpful. Time spent in preparing brief guidelines is worth the effort if they reinforce learning. It must be remembered, however, that handouts are supplemental and do not replace the need for class demonstration and supervised practice.

The provision of adequate, supervised practice can be a problem when a large group of employees is required to learn how to operate new equipment or how to perform a new procedure. In a large institution the staff development educator cannot personally supervise the practice of large numbers of learners. It is recommended that the supervision of practice be delegated to head nurses who will first be instructed by the staff development educator. This arrangement provides for shared responsibility and involves key unit nursing personnel in the development of their own staff members. If records of achievement are required, this, too, should be at the unit level, where those who still need practice can be identified and provided with opportunities to do so. This arrangement is recommended for any agency. Staff development is everyone's responsibility.

Self-instructional methods

Self-instructional methods are useful when a subject must be taught repeatedly; when learners can be allowed to set their own pace; or when instruction of staff members is needed at a time when the staff development educator is unavailable.

Programmed instruction. Although programmed instruction is time-consuming in its preparation and requires much material, it involves the student in self-learning and provides indications of progress and achievement.

Orientation to tasks involving either data, people, or things can be taught this way. Once developed, the lesson is available for all shifts and for new groups of employees, and it frequently provides a high yield of results in terms of learning. While some find this method of learning boring, most agree that they do learn. Many programmed instruction lessons are available commercially. At William Beaumont Hospital, several programmed instruction lessons have been designed and used for specific task orientation. One was developed to teach operating room technician trainees how to identify retractors. Cutout catalogue pictures of retractors were used throughout the lesson for identification purposes. The technician trainees learned to recognize the retractors, how to pronounce the names, and how they are used. Another programmed instruction lesson was developed to teach the principles of fire prevention, another to teach interpretation of electrocardiographs with regard to selected arrythmias. In the latter instance, a representative sample of electrocardiograph strips was collected and utilized to learn how to recognize certain arrhythmias (Fig. 9-4). The use of a new imprinter machine was also taught by programmed instruction. This was a "things" orientation where the learner was required to go to the machine and to use it as part of the lesson. The correct use was indicated by the imprint, which could be checked against the samples in the programmed lesson. Post-tests to check learning are either built into the lesson or provided as a follow-up check.

Slide-sound presentation. The slide-sound presentation involves a series of 35 mm slides and an audiotape that automatically advances the slide on prerecorded cues. Most audiovisual dealers can provide tape recorders with the attachments necessary for this type of presentation. Revision of content is easily accomplished by replacing slides. The principles of this presentation are much the same as those involved with *filmstrips, records,* or *cassette tapes.* However, it is difficult and expensive to prepare a filmstrip. Most self-

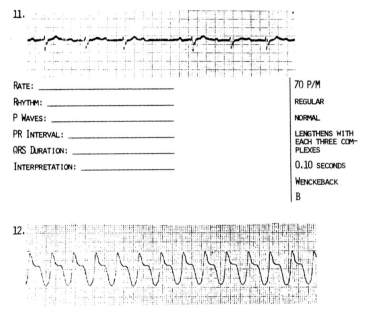

PAGE 17

USE CALIPERS TO GIVE THE FIVE FACTS NECESSARY TO IDENTIFY THE FOLLOWING AS FIRST OR SECOND DEGREE OR WENCKEBACK HEART BLOCKS. WRITE YOUR AN- SWERS IN THE BLANKS PROVIDED. FOR THOSE YOU FEEL ARE NOT 1°, 2°, WRITE NA IN THE INTERPRETATION BLANK. CONTINUE USE OF COVER STRIP ON ANSWER COLUMN.

11.

RATE: _____   70 P/M

RHYTHM: _____   REGULAR

P WAVES: _____   NORMAL

PR INTERVAL: _____   LENGTHENS WITH
                                     EACH THREE COM-
QRS DURATION: _____   PLEXES

INTERPRETATION: _____   0.10 SECONDS

                                     WENCKEBACK

                                     B

12.

Fig. 9-4. Sample page from a staff-designed programmed instruction lesson to provide opportunities to practice recognition of certain cardiac arrhythmias. (Courtesy William Beaumont Hospital, Royal Oak, Mich.)

instructional lessons presented by filmstrip are commercially prepared and may or may not suit the particular orientation purposes, since they tend to generalize the topic. Filmstrips and slide-sound materials may be used by an individual learner or a large group.

Short-cartridge super 8 movies. Short-cartridge super 8 movies can be used to orient one or more learners to a task. These movies are not difficult or expensive to prepare, are three minutes in length, and usually do not have sound. The lack of sound can be overcome by including an audiotape with the movie or preparing a viewing guide explain-

ing the key points of the presentation. The guide may be given to the viewer for later review. We have had particular success with one teaching cartridge on tracheostomy suctioning. The portability of equipment, the short lesson that is easily replaced, and the viewing guide have been useful for orientation of new employees, patients and their families, and for general purposes of review. (See Fig. 9-5.)

Audiotapes. Audiotapes can be used as a self-instructional approach. While audiotapes are easy to use, they share the limitations of the lecture. Once again, these faults can be

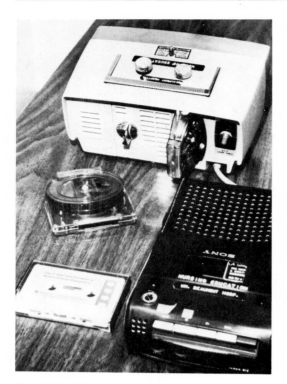

Fig. 9-5. Silent, cartridge loop film projector. Sound may be added through use of audiotape. (Courtesy William Beaumont Hospital, Royal Oak, Mich.)

overcome by providing an outline of the lecture points that will be available for future reference (Fig. 9-6).

Videotapes

Videotapes can be used for evaluation of task performance. Athletes have used this approach for some time to evaluate their performance in practice or during competition. We use videotape in the midterm examination for operating room technician trainees. The student technician is videotaped as he scrubs, gowns, sets up sterile tables and equipment, etc. The instructor and student then review the tape, as it provides a means for teaching and evaluation.[5]

UNIT ORIENTATION

There are a variety of ways to orient new employees to the nursing unit: the checklist of tasks to be learned, the buddy system, the do-it-yourself method, and internships. Much is written about orientation in terms of individualizing the experiences, starting at the level of the learner, and the special needs of today's new graduates.

If enough time were available, employees with preservice preparation eventually would attain their performance level capacity without the aid of orientation offerings. However, time is a highly costly commodity, and one of the objectives of a planned orientation program is to achieve optimum performance in a minimum of time. Another objective is to reduce and control the number of sources from which the new employee receives information. Regardless of past experience in other agencies, new employees need opportunities to practice in the new environment.

The concept discussed earlier, which proposes that any job (patient care, in this instance) is the sum of separate tasks, can be adapted to the design of a unit orientation. To apply this concept, it is necessary to identify and list the types of patients typically assigned to the unit. Tasks that comprise each type of patient care are also identified and added to the list. The list of patient categories and the tasks to be performed for each category are used as a guide for orientation assignments. Tasks are then integrated into the total care of the patient and not learned in a fragmented fashion as separate entities (Fig. 9-7).

When orientation experiences are organized in a patient-centered system, the competencies, skills, and knowledge that are demonstrated by the orientee provide a means to determine whether more or less orientation is needed.

To be a meaningful learning experience, standards of care must be identified clearly and discussed with the orientee along with each patient assignment. Details of the tasks to be performed must also be discussed. Maintenance of a record of orientation assignment, discussion, and level of competence in performance provides a means to measure orientation progress.

WILLIAM BEAUMONT HOSPITAL
DEPARTMENT OF NURSING EDUCATION

GUIDE TO CONTENT OF TAPE: LIABILITY AND THE NURSE

MR. MCGREGOR:

GENERAL POSITION OF HOSPITAL
RE LIABILITY

PERSONAL RESPONSIBILITY FOR OWN
NEGLIGENCE

CORPORATE FAULT

RESPONDEAT SUPERIOR

NURSES' LIABILITY:
O.R. NURSE - BORROWED SERVANT RULE

STANDARDS OF CARE

RESPONSIBILITY FOR OWN NEGLIGENCE

GOOD SAMARITAN LAW

LIABILITY INSURANCE

MR. ROBERTS:

SURGICAL CONSENT FORM

CRITERIA FOR VALID CONSENT

REQUIREMENTS FOR DOCUMENTING POST-OP
PROGRESS

REFUSAL OF BLOOD OR TREATMENT

AGE OF MAJORITY

GZ/CR
REVISED 10-72

Fig. 9-6. Topic outline to assist the listener to follow points in an audiotape presentation. (Courtesy William Beaumont Hospital, Royal Oak, Mich.)

5.

UNIT ORIENTATION PLAN AND PROGRESS RECORD
(CONTINUED)

UNIT: 4 NORTH

NAME_____ POSITION TITLE_____ DATE EMPLOYED_____

ASSIGNMENT TO: PATIENT CATEGORY OR ACTIVITY	PROVIDES EXPERIENCE IN OR KNOWLEDGE OF:	DISCUSSED (DATE AND INITIAL)	ASSIGNED DATE(S)	COMMENTS
PATIENT WITH IMPLANTED PACEMAKER	CHECKING APICAL AND RADIAL PULSE			
	RECOGNIZING SIGNS OF PACEMAKER MALFUNCTION			
	CARE OF WOUND SITE			
	PACEMAKER ARTIFACT ANALYSIS ROUTINE			
	PATIENT AND FAMILY TEACHING			
	ORIGINATING, IMPLEMENTING, UPDATING NURSING CARE PLAN			
PATIENT WITH EXTERNAL PACEMAKER	CHECKING APICAL AND RADIAL PULSES			
	CHECKING BATTERY FUNCTION			
	MAINTAINING ELECTRICAL SAFETY			
	OPERATION OF EXTERNAL POWER PACK:			
	CARE OF INSERTION SITE			
	RECOGNIZING SIGNS OF PACEMAKER FAILURE			
	PATIENT AND FAMILY TEACHING			
	ORIGINATING, IMPLEMENTING, UPDATING NURSING CARE PLAN			
PATIENT WITH CHRONIC DEBILITATING ILLNESS E.G., CVA, MALIGNANCY	SUPPORTIVE NURSING CARE			
	INTERDEPARTMENTAL RELATIONSHIPS:			
	PHYSICAL THERAPY, OCCUPATIONAL THERAPY, SPEECH THERAPY, SOCIAL SERVICE, HOME CARE			
	COMMUNICATING WITH TERMINALLY ILL PATIENT AND FAMILY			
	PATIENT AND FAMILY TEACHING			
	ORIGINATING, IMPLEMENTING, UPDATING NURSING CARE PLAN			

Fig. 9-7. Portion of a unit orientation assignment and progress record in which tasks to be learned are integrated into total patient care. (Courtesy William Beaumont Hospital, Royal Oak, Mich.)

SELECTION OF TEACHING METHODS FOR CONTINUING EDUCATION

Continuing education is concerned with increasing the competency of the employee. Attendance may be required or voluntary according to the policy of the agency or the priority of the content to be learned. The selection of a teaching method, as always, depends on the type of learner, the complexity of the material, and the availability of staff, resources, facilities, and materials. Continuing education may be presented in the form of seminars, workshops, lectures, panel discussions, short-term courses, nursing problem clinics, journal clubs, library study, etc.

Group process

The group process is the sine qua non of all instructional approaches when interaction of the participants is a major goal. Teaching methods utilizing a group process in one form or another are more often selected for continuing education activities than for orientation purposes. Conferences, workshops, seminars, journal clubs, and selected learning games usually include some form of the group process. Although varying labels are attached to teaching methods in which the group process is utilized, a basic structure is usually present. A leader is necessary to (1) introduce the topic, (2) define the purpose, (3) explain

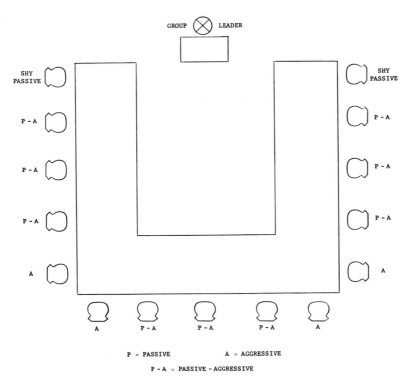

GROUP ⊗ LEADER

SHY PASSIVE

P - A

P - A

P - A

A

SHY PASSIVE

P - A

P - A

P - A

A

A P - A P - A P - A A

P = PASSIVE   A = AGGRESSIVE

P - A = PASSIVE - AGGRESSIVE

Fig. 9-8. U-shaped discussion group. Less aggressive group members can be drawn into the discussion when aggressive participants are seated farthest from the leader in the U-shaped group arrangement. (Courtesy William Beaumont Hospital, Royal Oak, Mich.)

the scope of discussion, (4) describe procedure, and (5) create a climate for the exchange of ideas. The extent of group control exercised by the leader depends on the desired goals and the ability of the group to achieve these goals.

Group size and seating arrangements are important aspects of group interaction. Ideally, a group should be kept to fifteen or less. When groups are larger than fifteen, physical distance alone can make communication difficult. Seating arrangements also affect the interchange of ideas among group members. The familiar circle of chairs or the round or square conference tables permit eye contact and face-to-face communication among all members. If a rectangular-shaped table is all that is available, members tend to be lined up along the sides and some members find it

difficult to communicate. When a rectangular table is used, the problem of involving all members can be overcome by placing the strong, aggressive members in the corner seats with the more passive members in between. In this way, less active participants tend to be drawn into the discussion. This presupposes that the leader knows the characteristics of the members in advance and requires a preestablished seating arrangement.

When the leader chooses to be in firm control of the group, such as in a discussion conducted through structured questions, a U-shaped table arrangement with the leader located at the open end is useful. To achieve a balance of interaction in the group, the members must be carefully placed according to their ability to participate. Passive members should be placed in closest contact with the leader, while aggressive members can be placed in the far corner seats (Fig. 9-8).

In any group process, proper facilities, techniques, and clearly identified directions help, but do not assure, the capability of the group to master communication problems among themselves. Often the success of the group in achieving its goals depends on the leader's ability to introduce the topic in such a way that it is understood and can be openly discussed without fear of reprisal either from the group or the leader. Everyone has an opinion and should be allowed to express it in a group discussion. The right to individual opinion is fundamental to the group process regardless of goal, topic, or selected teaching method.

Several instructional methods utilizing group process principles are included in this section. The approach may differ in each, but the basic principles of group process do not.

Workshop

A workshop provides an active learning experience for one or more groups who attempt to explore solutions to assigned topics or problems. Some orientation to the topic usually precedes the establishing of work groups. Speakers, videotapes, movies, case studies, etc. may be used to introduce the participants to the general workshop topic. Following this, the audience is then separated into small groups of five to seven people to develop solutions to specific assignments. Group leaders may be selected prior to the workshop and provided directions for guiding the work of their groups. This effort saves time and reduces communications problems that may exist if group members are not acquainted with each other. In the absence of a pre-assigned group leader, printed directions for assignments should be available. Directions should be short, clearly stated, and as simple as possible. When directions are lengthy and complicated, much time is lost in their translation and interpretation. The physical distance between groups should be such that one is not distracted by the conversation of

another. As in all group discussions, members should be seated to permit eye contact and adequate writing space should be provided. As an instructional method, the workshop is useful for continuing education purposes when participants need experience in group problem solving or when there is a need for group exploration of a single subject through utilization of information that has been presented.

Institute

Institutes differ from workshops since they tend to last longer, are somewhat more formal, and deal in long- rather than short-range goals. Both are valid continuing education activities. The institute involves a series of presentations by content specialists with little audience participation.[6] In order to involve the audience in active participation, some provision should be made for small groups to discuss selected aspects of the overall subject. Unlike the workshop, which generally has its focus on one central topic, the institute may cover several major areas. Since much of the presentation is in the form of lecture, the hazards of this method of teaching should be recalled. Again, it might be wise to provide topic outlines for each lecture. For continuing education purposes, the institute is advantageous when the learners have a need to acquire information about many aspects of one central subject.

Seminar

The seminar is an informal method in which the learners come prepared to discuss a specific topic. Initially, the subject may be presented by a content specialist or through a case study, a movie, etc. One or more learner-participants may present selected aspects of the topic, in which case the leader must be well informed in order to coordinate the discussion. An audience usually is not included. As in all group processes, the participants need to be seated in such a way as to make it possible to see each other. The seminar approach should be used when the continuing education needs are to acquire information on a special subject through utilization of a content specialist and through individual preseminar preparation. As an instructional approach, a series of seminars could be presented to staff members newly assigned to a specialized service. Since learner-participants are expected to study independently prior to the seminar, this method may produce a higher learning yield than other methods.

Panel discussion

The panel is a group discussion conducted before an audience. Prior to the discussion, each panel member makes a prepared presentation on some aspect of the general topic. An informal discussion among the panel follows. The leader-moderator coordinates the discussion but does not need to be a subject specialist because the panel is comprised of specialists. Members of the audience may participate by interjecting their personal views or by asking questions. On the whole, the audience tends to be passive and the retention of subject content limited. The panel members should be visible to each other as well as to the audience. This method is selected when interest in a general subject has been expressed and when increased competency of the staff is not the primary goal.

Nursing problem clinic

Nursing problem clinics, sometimes called grand rounds, can be useful for continuing education purposes as they provide opportunities for members of a nursing staff to work through a particularly difficult nursing care problem with other nursing staff personnel. It is recommended that the steps of the nursing process be utilized to organize the presentation—assessment, planning, implementation, and evaluation.° Needs that were identified,

° A singularly commendable synthesis of the recipient-centered nursing process is available in the pamphlet *Position on Nursing Practice,* distributed by the Michigan Nurses' Association, East Lansing, Mich.

plans that were developed and implemented, and the evaluation of results are shared with others in the nursing problem clinic. At the William Beaumont Hospital the presentation is recorded on videotape and then shown on closed-circuit television according to a prearranged schedule. The television viewers are invited to complete a critique in which they indicate whether all needs were identified satisfactorily and whether they agreed with the solutions. The critiques completed by the audience are then shared with the staff who presented the clinic. Opportunities for both self- and peer-evaluations are entailed in this teaching approach.

Journal club

The formation of a journal club is one way to provide opportunities for discussion of subjects that appear in recent periodicals or journals. As a rule, the group has a commitment to meet on a regular basis even though its membership is voluntary. The discussion format can be whatever the group wishes it to be. One member may volunteer to read and report on an article, or all may choose to study the article with a volunteer acting as discussion coordinator. The group should ultimately be self-directed, although it may require some initial assistance in working out the details.

Conference

The conference, another instructional method utilizing the principles of group process, usually involves the discussion of a specific problem. Conducted somewhat formally, its goal is to identify the solutions to a problem. Participants might be confined to the unit members of a nursing staff who seek the answer to a particular nursing or patient care problem. The conference may also involve members from several units who are experiencing similar problems. Whatever the case, the group leader must be knowledgeable of group process techniques in order to effectively utilize the contributions of the group members.

Short-term course

Short-term courses in a staff development program provide selected staff members the opportunity to increase their competency in a special nursing or patient care area. Courses such as acute coronary care, medication administration, and management of patient care are examples of short-term courses that expand the knowledge and skills of the learner. As a rule, most participants come to the course with limited knowledge or skill in the subject, acquired either in preservice education or through work experience. The multimedia approach, which utilizes a variety of audiovisual aids to present content, may be selected for short courses. There are some advantages to the multimedia system. Audiotapes, cartridge movies, filmstrips, videotapes, and programmed instruction may be available to those who miss class or need to repeat the information. Some of the audiovisual information may be used for orientation or single continuing education classes. Disadvantages of the multimedia approach include the costs for both hardware and software and the class disorganization that occurs if the projection equipment breaks down or the software is misplaced. The staff development educator must be adaptable as well as knowledgeable about the subject matter in order to teach without aids when necessary. Some record of short-term course participation should be maintained in the participant's personnel file.

Learning game

Learning games for continuing education follow specific rules, present some type of challenge, may be competitive in nature, and can be viewed as a form of play activity through which learning takes place. Role play, in-basket exercise, Pigors' incident process, and crossword puzzles are a few examples of learning games or simulation exercises.

Role play. Through the simulation of real-life characters and situations, role play can be used to illustrate a point or to provide individuals with insight into another's viewpoint or position. If emotional reactions are un-

checked and controls and restrictions are not imposed, role playing can be an unpleasant experience for participants and audience alike. Roles to be played and some general ground rules must be clearly identified prior to the event. The need to "de-role" the participants at the end of the performance is nicely brought out by Cooper and Hornback.[7] They recommend that the players be applauded or asked to make the first comments so that the termination of the role play is clearly marked.

In-basket exercise. The in-basket exercise is a popular way to acquire skill in decision making and problem identification. In this exercise the contents of the basket (mailbox) are assigned priority and the appropriate actions are decided by the participants. Like role play, this game is designed to place participants in positions where they encounter problems usually faced by those in other positions. The Hospital Research and Educational Trust has an inexpensive, nicely organized in-basket exercise called, "You Are Barbara Jordan." Twenty-five mailbox communications, notes, letters, directives, etc. are included in this basket that the student, now Barbara Jordan, must dispose of in one way or another. Materials for this exercise are inexpensive and well organized.[*] At the William Beaumont Hospital, a course for staff nurses has been designed in which the principles of management are applied to the care of patients. The concept of the in-basket exercise was adapted to the course by using the mailbox folder containing simulated contents of the head nurse's mailbox to provide an orientation to one of the head nurse's tasks and roles. Contents are assorted and categorized according to functional areas such as staffing, patient care, staff development, communication, and budget, and actions to be taken are identified (Fig. 9-9).

Pigors' incident process. The Pigors' incident process is another game approach

[*]"You Are Barbara Jordan" in-basket exercise kits are available from Hospital Research and Educational Trust, 40 North Lake Shore Drive, Chicago, Ill.

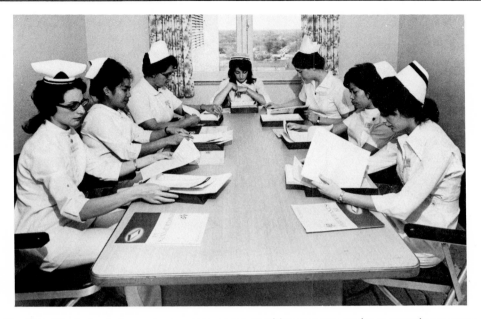

Fig. 9-9. The in-basket exercise learning game provides an opportunity to experience someone else's role. (Courtesy William Beaumont Hospital, Royal Oak, Mich.)

that can be used as a problem-solving learning experience.[8] This is used best in groups of twelve to sixteen. The object is to ask questions that bring to light the facts involved in the hypothetical incident and to determine the most relevant question. "Was the supervisor justified . . . ?" "Should the OR nurse have refused . . . ?" The questions should require only yes or no answers. All participants are required to commit themselves to an answer. The "yes" group separates from the "no" group. All group members must be able to justify their response. A spokesman selected from each group defends his group's position in a debate. The success of the process depends on the selection of an incident that is controversial and has a two-way pull. Learning takes place in the fact-finding period and in the debate. A series of these classes provides practice in asking relevant questions necessary for the identification of key issues involved in the incidents. This method is useful for all levels of employees. Nurse assistants who

are careless with patients' belongings, nurses who divide drug doses, and ward clerks who neglect to change dates on the imprinter at midnight are a few of the "incidents" that we have used for continuing education purposes (Fig. 9-10).

Crossword puzzle. Puzzles are popular with the staff and can provide a way to review material or to introduce new information. Crossword puzzles on the principles of dialysis were designed by the nurses on the hemodialysis unit and distributed to the general nursing staff as well as to the dialysis patients. The obstetrics staff designed a crossword puzzle on obstetrical nursing care; it was distributed to the general nursing staff and used by newly employed obstetrical staff nurses as part of their orientation. A puzzle on the subject of medical terminology, written by the unit clerk staff development educator, is used in training classes to teach new words and to review old ones. A puzzle devoted to the maintenance of fluid and electrolyte balance was distributed in

WILLIAM BEAUMONT HOSPITAL
DEPARTMENT OF NURSING EDUCATION

THE CASE OF THE DIVIDED DRUG DOSE

INCIDENT: ON AUGUST 11 AT 9:00 AM, MRS. WHIPPLE, A PATIENT WHO HAD A LEFT
UPPER LOBECTOMY TWO DAYS PREVIOUSLY, COMPLAINED TO DR. BROWN
THAT SHE HAD LITTLE OR NO RELIEF FROM HER MEDICATION. UPON
READING MRS. WHIPPLE'S CHART, DR. BROWN DISCOVERED SHE RECEIVED 50
MGM. OF DEMEROL AT 2:00 AM. TURNING TO THE HEAD NURSE, HE SAID,
"I'M GOING TO REPORT THIS MATTER TO THE NURSING OFFICE."

THE INCIDENT PROCESS:

    I.   THE INCIDENT

    II.   THE FACTS

        A.   SCENE AND SEQUENCE OF ACTION
        B.   THE DETAILS — WHAT, WHEN, WHERE, HOW, WHO
        C.   THE FACTS SUMMARIZED

    III.   WHAT NEEDS TO BE DECIDED?

        A.   WHAT IS THE QUESTION?
        B.   ARE THERE SUB-QUESTIONS?

    IV.   THE DECISION

        A.   CHOOSE AN ANSWER TO THE MAIN QUESTION
        B.   WHAT IS YOUR REASONING?

    V.   THE BROADER ISSUE

        A.   WHAT IS AT STAKE?
        B.   WHAT CAN BE LEARNED?

DHC/CJR
8-8-68

Fig. 9-10. Sample incident used in the incident process learning game. (Courtesy William Beaumont Hospital, Royal Oak, Mich.)

the *Nursing Education Newsletter*° following a review seminar on the principles of fluid and electrolyte balance.

TYPES OF SETTINGS AND PLANNING GUIDE

An illustration of seating arrangements for some typical group activities is found in Fig. 9-11. A planning guide for selecting an appropriate room size and seating plan is found in Table 9-1.

SELECTION OF TEACHING AIDS

The selection of an appropriate teaching aid requires some familiarity with the capabilities and limitations of both hardware (equipment) and software (the message). With

°William Beaumont Hospital inhouse nursing publication.

the proliferation and wide cost range of audio-visual materials, the choice of an economical teaching aid has become more difficult. Selection is influenced by budget restrictions, by the department's philosophy and program, and by specific learning objectives. Budget restrictions, for obvious reasons, definitely influence the choice. Whether to use commercially prepared software or to develop it within the agency is a consideration in the choice of hardware that involves both budget and philosophy.

It should be remembered that acquisition of hardware does not solve learning needs—a teaching aid is a supplement, not a substitute. It is also important to remember that the budget appropriation for hardware must include provision for the continuing cost of software.

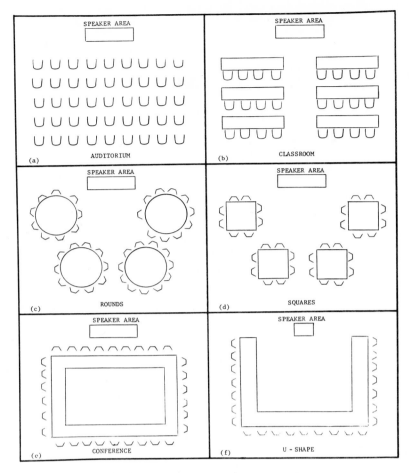

Fig. 9-11. Group seating arrangements. **a,** Auditorium. **b,** Classroom. **c,** Rounds (tables or chairs). **d,** Squares (tables or chairs). **e,** Conference. **f,** U-shaped conference. See Table 9-1 for a guide to select settings. (Courtesy William Beaumont Hospital, Royal Oak, Mich.)

Table 9-1. Guide for planning settings

Purpose of offering	Method	Setting
Information giving	Lecture Panel Institute Self-instruction	Auditorium Classroom Carrel
Problem solving	Seminar Conference Case study Learning games Self-instruction	Conference Rounds Squares Carrel
Skill development (procedures, equipment, directing others)	Lecture with demonstration Return demonstration Learning games Self-instruction	Small auditorium Classroom Conference Carrel

A sophisticated piece of hardware is of little value if there is no continuing provision to acquire software.

Whether to use commercially prepared software or to "do it yourself" depends on the department's philosophy and objectives. Does the philosophy require that the staff be involved in its own learning? If so, one way is to utilize the talents of the staff in the production of relevant teaching aids for staff development or for patient education. Does the commercially prepared software do a better job for you? Most software is of technically good quality, and much of it is prepared by content specialists. However, it is also expensive.

Some of the usual teaching aids are discussed in this section. Major features, limitations, relative costs, and some uses are described. Discussion of aids is separated into the categories of audio, visual, and audiovisual.

Audio

Tape recorders that play either reel-to-reel or cartridge tapes are the principal auditory aids. All audiotape is erasable, can be reused, and is inexpensive. However, as has been mentioned previously, an aid that involves only the auditory sense requires supplementation such as the printed topic outline. Topic outlines provide a visual aid and make it easier to follow the content.

Reel-to-reel tape recorders. Some characteristics of the reel-to-reel tape recorder are that it usually has several recording speeds, requires hand threading, is larger than the cartridge tape recorder, and as a rule requires a direct electrical power source. Many can be used as an amplifier loudspeaker as well.

Compared to the cartridge tape recorder, the reel-to-reel recorder is less portable, costs more, and is more difficult to thread. However, its sound has better quality and the available recording time is greater than that of the smaller cartridge tape recorder. Because the volume is good, this recorder can be used for large audiences and can be connected to the microphone system.

Cartridge tape recorders. Recorders that use cartridge tape vary in model and cost. The attractive features of a cartridge tape recorder are the ease with which it is operated and its portability. Many recorders are available with built-in microphones and can be powered by battery as well as direct electric current.

Cartridge tape is inexpensive and the recording time varies from fifteen minutes to two hours. It has been our experience that the longer tapes tend to provide less sound fidelity and become tangled in the cartridge more often than the shorter tapes. Also, the shorter (therefore thicker) tape appears to be more reusable. Cartridge tape recorders are limited primarily to small group use. Because of the portability of the recorder, it is possible to record speeches, meetings, question and answer periods, case studies, and lectures. It is recommended that topics of special value be copied and the original retained in a safe place. A second recorder and an inexpensive jack cord are required for this purpose (Fig. 9-12). Valuable content can be locked into place by removing a small plastic tab located directly above the letter on the label indicating the side of the tape. Accidental erasure of content is avoided by removing this tab. Wider distribution and increased use of tapes is possible when extra copies are available.

Video

Filmstrips, super 8 loop films, 35 mm slides, and transparencies are some of the familiar visual teaching aids. The required hardware is easy to operate, fairly inexpensive, and portable. Electric power, a viewing screen, and a darkened room are required for most equipment of this kind.

Commercially prepared video software has good technical quality on the whole. Subject specialists are frequently consulted in producing the content. Costs for software vary widely; some software is available at no cost from pharmaceutical companies, while others may be very costly considering the short message presented. In many instances, software for video use can be produced by staff devel-

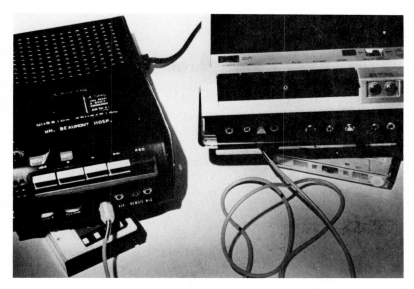

Fig. 9-12. Components for copying audiotapes. (Courtesy William Beaumont Hospital, Royal Oak, Mich.)

opment educators to meet learning needs specific to the nursing staff within the agency.

As with all teaching aids that are directed to only one sense, it is recommended that a viewing guide be produced and distributed to each viewer for subsequent review and reference.

Filmstrips. Filmstrips are compact, easy to store, thread easily into portable projectors, and can be used for small or large audiences. Most projectors are standard and can be used for all filmstrips. Projectors of all prices are available. Possible sound attachments include record and cassette-playing equipment designed to advance the filmstrip on electronic cue. As with most commercially prepared software, filmstrips have good technical quality. However, the quality of the content depends on its source. Costs of production are high, a fact reflected by the price per filmstrip. Thus long-range use should be anticipated when purchasing filmstrips. Filmstrips also are difficult and expensive for the staff development educator to produce. Loop films, 35 mm slides, and transparencies can be produced more easily and economically.

Super 8 loop films. Super 8 loop films come in cartridges and are shown with portable, easy to operate projectors. For the most part, films are silent and confined to three- or four-minute messages. The loop film was first known as single-concept film since the limited film time could include no more than one idea. Loop film is available today in longer length and with sound. Several types of projectors are available. Each, however, requires a different type of cartridge and one is not interchangeable with another. Therefore caution must be exercised in selecting the basic hardware.

Many commercially prepared loop films are available at reasonable cost. It is also possible to produce inexpensive loop films using super 8 home movie–type equipment. Cartridge-loading service is available or blank cartridges can be obtained and loaded at the agency. The problem with "home" production is that unless a perfectly executed performance can be shot without pause, the film must be edited and spliced. Splices tend to break if the film is used a great deal. Loop films have many attractive features, including low cost, easy operation, and portability to treatment rooms, patients' bedsides, and small conference rooms. To overcome the lack of sound, it is recommended that a small printed guide to viewing be available for study prior to watching the film as well as for later reference. Audiotapes can be prepared to accompany the film, but the amateur operator may have difficulty synchronizing the audio with the visual aspect of the lesson. These films can be used by an individual or by small groups and are excellent teaching aids for reviewing infrequently used procedures.

Thirty-five–millimeter slides. The 35 mm color slide is an inexpensive, versatile teaching aid that can be used with both small and large audiences to illustrate lecture points, teach procedures, or provide titles for videotapes. Although some slides are available commercially, staff development educators can easily and inexpensively produce slide presentations that are oriented to their specific learning need. While most slides are permanent, there are title slides available on which a message or illustration can be hand drawn or typed and later erased for reuse. Although slides are still pictures, it is possible to simulate action by showing a series of slides quickly, starting with an overall shot and moving slide by slide to a tight closeup. This also can be accomplished by using several projectors to show three or more slides in quick sequence on the same screen. This type of presentation, while effective, is difficult to organize and operation of the equipment can be confusing to the amateur.

Slide projectors have been standardized and are easy to operate. Inexpensive models to fairly expensive and highly versatile equipment can be selected. Preview capability, automatic focus, timing devices, and adaptors for automatic advance on sound cues from recorders are a few of the attractive features of the newer, more expensive models.

Since slides are easily separated and lost, it is recommended that frequently used slides be stored in slide trays or carousels. Slide trays are inexpensive and store easily but do not hold as many slides as the carousel. If many slide presentations are anticipated, it is recommended that a projector that accepts both tray and carousel be considered.

Transparencies. As a teaching aid, the flat transparency is used mainly to illustrate a lecture or to guide a discussion by projecting data, printed material, or illustrations onto a screen by way of an overhead projector. While some transparencies are available commercially, many staff development educators make their own. Construction materials for creating professional-looking transparencies are available from art and audiovisual distributors. Additionally, certain copying machines will copy material onto blank transparencies quite well. Rolls of blank transparency material are available, making it possible to develop illustrations or data to be presented that can be rolled through the projector in sequence.

Overhead projectors through which the transparency message is projected are rather large but lightweight, portable, and not too expensive. Transparencies can be used in the same way as a chalkboard except that the lecturer remains facing the audience while using the overhead projector. Another advantage of transparencies over the chalkboard is that the transparencies may be retained for future use. This teaching aid can be used for small or large audiences but is not well suited to self-instruction.

Bulletin boards. While bulletin boards obviously do not fall into the category of power-driven teaching aids, they should be included as useful visual aids. This can be one of the least expensive tools. An economy-minded staff development educator collects illustrations, colored paper from magazines, and advertisements for future bulletin board use. Reusable letters, inexpensive wallboard, and a few art store books on preparing effective bulletin boards should be added to the collection. Examples of good design and professionally prepared messages that might be adapted to a particular need are available in every magazine.

Bulletin boards can be a complete lesson or

can complement a current staff development project. One particularly effective teaching bulletin board that serves both purposes was used as an adjunct to a series of lectures on epilepsy. A bulletin board was prepared with the title "'What is Your EQ? (Epilepsy Quotient)," below which were four brief questions. Four folded papers containing the answers were attached along the lower edge of the board. After a week, the dog-eared answer papers were a testimonial to the fact that it did attract readers.

A few brief hints can be offered here. Location is important. For example, the bulletin board on epilepsy was located in the locker room lounge. The board would have been less effective had it been placed in a spot where traffic did not stop. Only the briefest of content can be placed in busy locations. More involved messages may be placed near a cafeteria line and in lounges, classrooms, or conference rooms. A portable bulletin board display could be rotated through the units on a shared basis. Most of us are lazy readers and want instant messages. We also need some type of "come-on" in the form of a point of interest that attracts us to the message. Color coordination can attract us to the display as well as tie the points together. Examples of these techniques can be found in most magazines. One final suggestion is to replace the bulletin board display often. Even the most effective bulletin boards hold staff interest for only a short time.

Audiovisual

Audiovisual hardware and software include the best of two worlds since both sound and sight are involved. The most commonly used audiovisuals are the 16 mm movies, the 35 mm slide-sound, filmstrips with sound, and television. A newcomer to the audiovisual teaching aid group is the sound-page.

Commercially prepared audiovisual software has good technical quality. With both audio and visual senses involved, it is always a temptation to tailor the lesson to fit the audiovisual message rather than to use it as an aid to reach a preplanned objective. As always, the objectives and philosophy as well as the budget determine the choice of audiovisual hardware and software.

Sixteen-millimeter movies. The 16 mm movie is one of the most familiar teaching aids. High quality of color and sound is a feature of 16 mm movies. The films vary in length from short discussion-starters to full-length, 40- to 60-minute reels. Because the cost of producing a movie is very high, the films are quite expensive. Most staff development educators rent or purchase films rather than produce their own. Rental fees are reasonable, but availability of showing dates does not always coincide with schedules and program plans. A viewing screen and space adequate for focus and picture size are required, as is a darkened room. The 16 mm movies can be used for large or small audiences. Since the operation of the equipment requires some skill, the 16 mm movie is not often used for self-instruction.

Most 16 mm film is available in reel-to-reel form and can be used interchangeably on all reel-type projectors, whether hand-threaded or automatic. Costs for projectors range widely but can be assumed to be expensive.

Thirty-five–millimeter slide-sound. In the slide-sound technique, the message is recorded on audiotape and accompanying slides further illustrate each point. Special equipment is required; the tape recorder must be equipped to record electronic slide-advance cues on the audiotape at each point where the slide needs to be advanced. Most slide projectors are built to accept a special jack wire that attaches to the audiotape recorder and through which the advance cues are received.

All the advantages offered by slide presentations are available in slide-sound. Audiotape is easily erased and reused, and single slides are easy to replace. Equipment for slide-sound presentations is not inexpensive, but the cost is made up for by its versality. This type of aid is best for small to average-size groups or for self-instruction.

Filmstrips with sound. Principles of the use of filmstrips with sound as a teaching aid are much the same as for the 35 mm slide-sound approach. However, while single, separate slides can be lost, the filmstrip pictures are attached in a continuous roll. On the other hand, revisions in content are easier when slides are used, as they are easy to replace. This is not possible with filmstrips. Filmstrip is also more expensive than slides. Costs for projectors are also moderately higher. Sound for filmstrips is available in disk record or cartridge audiotape. In either case, recorded cues advance the picture frame at the appropriate point. Many commercial products record silent advance cues on one side of the record or audiotape for automatic advance, while the opposite side has audible sound signals for manual advance should automatic equipment not be available. Viewing guides usually accompany commercially prepared sound-filmstrip materials.

Costs for software may or may not be high, depending on the long-range use to which it is put. If cardiopulmonary resuscitation is taught fifty-two weeks a year, the cost for a sound-filmstrip that does a good job of illustrating the points to be learned is not high.

Sound-page. One of the newer audiovisual teaching aids is the sound-page. The software is an 8 × 11 inch page that has a magnetized back on which four minutes of sound can be recorded in a strictly do-it-yourself manner. The small portable machine uses the same needle to record and play back the four-minute message. Each sheet costs approximately 30 cents. Procedures, illustrations, points of discussion, photographs, or whatever is indicated can be attached to or drawn on the opposite side of the page. The four minutes of discussion refers to the illustrations. The sound has true fidelity and the volume is especially good. An electric erasing device is available at a small cost, making it possible to reuse the sheets if desired. In essence, the page literally talks to the learner who is operating the machine. Pages must be placed and turned by hand. Some patients may need help with this procedure. It is best used for one or two learners because viewing the illustrated page would be difficult for more than two.

One example of the use of the sound-page can be cited. Nurses in the kidney unit prepared a lesson to teach patients shunt care at

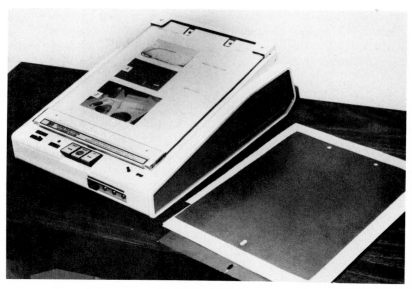

Fig. 9-13. Sound-page equipment. (Courtesy William Beaumont Hospital, Royal Oak, Mich.)

home. Photographs of the procedure were attached to two pages. An explanation of the procedure was recorded on the magnetized side of each page. A short pencil-and-paper, multiple-choice test was completed by the patient at the end of the lesson. Answers to the test were discussed on the third sound-page. Because patients are dialyzed for six hours at a time, this approach offers them a way to use their in-hospital time to good advantage. This same lesson is used by nurses on other units when they care for patients who have arteriovenous shunts. (See Fig. 9-13.)

TELEVISION

Television, as a medium of entertainment and source of information, has become a way of life for most of us. As a teaching aid, there are both advantages and disadvantages, but the weight is heavily on the side of the advantages. Certainly one of the most useful features of videotape is *image memory:* a videotaped lesson, lecture, or demonstration may be presented to any number of people at any time. Instant playback, a feature of many sports broadcasts, is possible through videotape and can be used to check procedure, performance, or lecture quality.

Another advantage provided by videotape is that of *image transportation,* by which it is possible for learners to have access to otherwise inaccessible locations. A classic example of the advantages of television and videotape is in operating rooms. Amphitheaters have been almost totally abandoned as a result.

Another advantage is *image association,* requiring two cameras and the switching of equipment but providing the advantage of a double image. For example, it is possible to record both the patient and the care plan in one view or, for use in a coronary care course, a patient and his electrocardiograph recording.

One of the special advantages of television and videotape is that it provides a way for individuals to be involved in their own learning. An example of this was mentioned earlier regarding the use of videotape for nursing problems clinics.

There are disadvantages as well as advantages to television as a teaching aid. One disadvantage is that TV does not stop to answer questions. Stop points and personal contact with the staff development educator may need to be built in. Cost of equipment is fairly high and beyond the means of some staff development departments. Costs of videotape must be considered also. Purchase cost for ½-inch black and white videotape ranges from 50 cents to one dollar a minute. However, videotape, like audiotape, can be erased and is available for several lessons, thus reducing the cost per lesson. A disadvantage presents itself in the actual operation of the playback videotape recorder—skill is required to operate the equipment. Although there is little problem with cartridge or cassette videotape, reel-to-reel videotape is easily destroyed by amateur operators. Another disadvantage is the high cost of color cameras, meaning that black and white videotape is used by most. In some instances, black and white is not so effective as color in illustrating a point.

The use of a story board to prepare scripts for TV, slides, or movies is useful for organizing approaches and visualizing the end results. The story board consists of a sheet of paper with blank squares and accompanying comment space. Stick figures or approximate representations of procedures or equipment are sketched into each square in sequence. Explanation of the sketch appears at the side as a guide to the cameraman (Fig. 9-14).

One major distinction can be made between live or taped closed-circuit television and the other audiovisual presentations. While movies, filmstrips, slides, loop films, and audiotapes are essentially limited to use in a single place, closed-circuit TV can be shown simultaneously in many locations, thus relieving some of the space and schedule problems.

Television offers many opportunities for the involvement of a staff in its own learning. Today's staff development educator in large institutions no longer can be the complete content specialist in all fields of nursing. Nursing staff members who are assigned to the

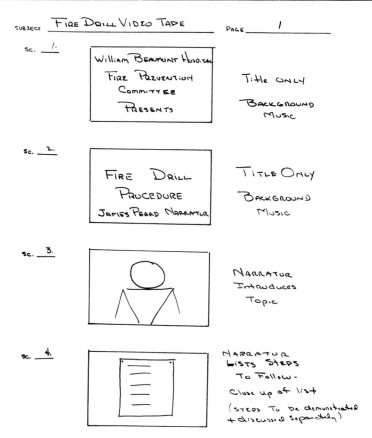

SUBJECT　Fire Drill Video Tape　PAGE　1

Sc. 1.

William Beaumont Hospital
Fire Prevention
Committee
Presents

Title Only

Background
Music

Sc. 2.

Fire　Drill
Procedure
James Peard Narrator

Title Only

Background
Music

Sc. 3.

Narrator
Introduces
Topic

Sc. 4.

Narrator
Lists Steps
To Follow —
Close up of list
(Steps To be demonstrated
+ discussed separately)

Fig. 9-14. Story board serves as a blueprint for developing television presentation. (Courtesy William Beaumont Hospital, Royal Oak, Mich.)

units become subject specialists in their own right. Opportunities to share their knowledge with others through videotaped demonstrations and discussions is a highly effective way to achieve competency through staff development. (See Fig. 9-15.)

AUDIOVISUAL COOPERATIVE GROUPS

Many references to the cost of teaching aids have been made in this chapter. In some areas, hospitals have formed audiovisual cooperatives to reduce costs by sharing available software, hardware, and talent. One audiovisual cooperative has compiled an annotated catalogue of members' hardware and software, including 300 films, slides, videotapes, transparencies, and audiotapes as well as an inventory of audiovisual equipment ranging from simple flip charts to complete multicamera, closed-circuit television systems. The membership of the cooperative includes artists, photographers, script writers, content specialists, and television cameramen.[9] There are many advantages to this approach, not the least of which are the opportunities to share mutual problems, materials, and the diverse skills of the members.

CONCLUSION

Selected appropriately, with concern for economy of time, material, and effort, the instructional aid can provide rewarding experiences for both teacher and learner, as long as the aid is fitted to the learning objective.

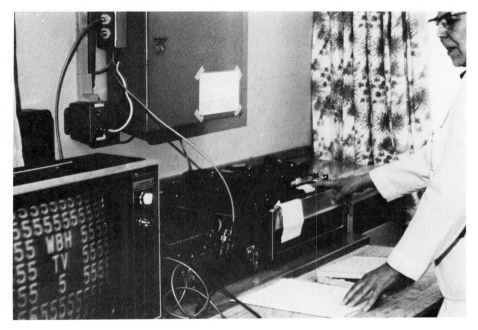

Fig. 9-15. Closed-circuit television system equipment includes videotape recorder, monitor, and sound and video amplification equipment. (Courtesy William Beaumont Hospital, Royal Oak, Mich.)

As was said at the beginning of this chapter, "... in the end it is the learner who must do the learning, and no amount of communication by lecture, by book, by film, by radio or by television will make the slightest difference unless he does something with what he receives."

REFERENCES

1. Coye, D. H.: The what of continuing education, Supervisor Nurse 1(11):37, 1970.
2. Coye, D. H.: Programmed instruction for staff education, Am. J. Nurs. 69:327, 1969.
3. Cantor, M.: Standard V—education for quality care, J. Nurs. Admin. 3(1):54, 1973.
4. Bernotavicz, F. D., and Wallington, J.: Act I of JIMS, Audiovis. Instr. 15:25, May, 1970.
5. Videotape recorder installed at Beaumont, Mich. Hosp. 6:27, Sept., 1970.
6. Hannigan, J. A.: The short term institute: a vehicle for continuing education, School Media Q. 1:193, Spring, 1973.
7. Cooper, S. S., and Hornback, M. S.: Continuing nursing education, New York, 1973, McGraw-Hill Book Co.
8. Pigors, P., Pigors, F., and Tribou, M.: Professional nursing practice: cases and issues, New York, 1967, McGraw-Hill Book Co.
9. Audiovisual cooperative established, Mich. Hosp. 8:23, Nov., 1972.

BIBLIOGRAPHY

American Management Association: Conference leadership manual, New York, 1965, The Association.
Boguslawski, M., and Judkins, B.: Contemporary guidelines in teaching, J. Nurs. Educ. 10(1):3, 1971.
Brylski, E., and Gilıen, E.: Audiovisuals made to order, Nurs. Outlook 20:385, 1972.
Crandall, G. M.: Videotape keeps the training up to date, holds the cost down, Mod. Hosp. 117(1):85, 1971.
Evaluating programmed instruction, Health Educ. Resources 2(7):126, 1972.
Hight, W. C.: A guide to A-V software, In-Serv. Train. Educ. 2:65, Jan.-Feb., 1973.
Hight, W. C.: A-V from A to Z, an equipment primer, In-Serv. Train. Educ. 1:96, Nov., 1972.
Homemade slide tapes are a bargain, but . . . , In-Serv. Train. Educ. 2:49, Jan.-Feb., 1973.
Hospitals use new technology of training to teach new technology of care, Mod. Hosp. 117(1):83, 1971.
In-Service education source book, Chicago, 1972, Modern Hospital Press.

Jamron, K. S., and Nailen, R. L.: Homemade videotapes train staff and help patients understand hospital procedures, Mod. Hosp. 117(1):87, 1971.

Mager, R. F.: Preparing objectives for programmed instruction, San Francisco, 1962, Fearon Publishers.

Marson, S. N.: Programmed instruction—panacea or passing gimmick? Int. Nurs. Rev. 19(2):126, 1972.

Mathis, R. L.: Learning theory and staff training, Supervisor Nurse 4(3):9, 1973.

Moore, M.: Staff development for the professional in the nursing service department, J. Cont. Educ. Nurs. 1(3):26, 1970.

Morgan, D. M.: Continuing education and staff development in hospitals, Can. Hosp. 49:35, Nov., 1972.

Niebel, H. H.: Single subject films—a new concept in continuing education, Milit. Med. 16:45, May, 1971.

Peterson, C. J.: Multisensory tutorial instruction in associate degree nursing education, Audiovis. Instr. 4:16, Feb., 1972.

Redman, B. K.: The process of patient teaching in nursing, ed. 2, St. Louis, 1972, The C. V. Mosby Co.

Rueschlaub, E. L.: Audiovisual self teaching aids can bolster inservice programs, Hosp. Topics 47(10):38, 1969.

Selected references on programmed instruction, Washington, D. C., Office of Education and Training. U. S. Department of Health, Education and Welfare.

Set goals then ask: did I get there? In-Serv. Train. Educ. 1:60, Nov., 1962.

Skinner, G.: What do practicing nurses want to know? Am. J. Nurs. 69:1662, 1969.

Smylie, H.: From nurse-teacher to audiovisual advisor, Can. Nurs. 68(10):29, 1972.

Svagr, V.: Introduction to programmed instruction, Pontiac, Mich., 1969, Reading and Language Center, Oakland Schools.

Taber, J. I., Glaser, R., and Schaefer, H. H.: Learning and programmed instruction, New York, 1965, Addison-Wesley Publishing Co., Inc.

Tobin, H. M., and Wengerd, J. S.: What makes a staff development program work? Am. J. Nurs. 71:940, 1971.

Truman, D. B.: The governmental process, New York, 1957, Alfred A. Knopf, Inc.

Wittmeyer, A.: Teaching by audiotape, Nurs. Outlook 19:162, 1971.

Wooley, A. S.: Reaching and teaching the older student, Nurs. Outlook 21:37, 1973.

Young, K.: Social psychology, New York, 1956, Appleton-Century-Crofts.

10

Evaluation

. . . evaluation is not merely a collection of techniques—evaluation is a process . . . .°

In preceding chapters it has been stated that evaluation should take place throughout the staff development process. It is generally agreed that learning brings about change in behavior. As cited in Fig. 1-2 (p. 5), change in behavior (performance behavior) is the end result of the staff development process. In the past, evaluation was not properly used to determine if change in behavior had occurred and, if so, to what degree the change was a result of staff development efforts. Without evaluation as an essential part of the process, it may never be known whether or why a particular offering is effective. In addition to standards that cite evaluation as an integral part of the overall staff development effort, concern with cost effectiveness and the need to justify expenditures necessitate evaluation. Consumers want their money used in appropriate and beneficial ways.

Evaluation also gives direction to planned changes by providing a base of facts rather than experiential or authoritative opinion. Finally, evaluation benefits the employees not only in terms of their output from a designated learning offering but also in terms of personal and professional development. Although many people view evaluation in a negative light, it frequently encourages the individual to adhere to an acceptable behavior or goal. If reinforcement or redirection through evaluation is not made, the individual may behave inappropriately simply because

he does not perceive his behavior as being unacceptable.

Hence staff development educators need to acquire a base of valid, reliable information. To establish this base, a system for collecting, organizing, analyzing, reporting, and acting must be designed.[1]

DEFINITION AND PURPOSE OF EVALUATION

Evaluation is the process of ascertaining or appraising the value of something. In staff development, evaluation is aimed at determining the value of specific learning offerings and the effectiveness of the overall effort. Evaluation differs from measurement. While evaluation ascribes worth or value, measurement documents quantity.

Measurements include a variety of testing procedures that describe output in quantitative terms. For example, it may be desirable to give a written test on the content covered in a particular course. The test results, whether percentage scores or letter grades, indicate how well given individuals "measured" against a predetermined standard of performance. Evaluation may include such test results as well as other quantitative and qualitative considerations. For example, it may be decided that the learners must (1) achieve certain test scores, (2) demonstrate their new knowledge in the clinical area, and (3) express the desirability for using the new knowledge in predetermined ways. Thus, in evaluation, consideration must be given to the type of data being analyzed. In some situations it may be important to weigh one aspect more heavily

°Gronlund, N. E.: Measurement and evaluation in teaching, New York, 1971, Macmillan Publishing Co., Inc.

than another in arriving at a value judgment; for example, using the knowledge may be more significant than identifying it. Once the documentation is made with facts, the judgment should be recorded and the learner must be informed of the evaluation results. In some situations, however, the learner is involved in the development of the evaluation.

As seen in Fig. 1-2, only evaluation has arrows emanating to all other phases of the staff development process, signifying its continual involvement. Although we have said that the various phases are interrelated and may be changed at any point in the process, evaluation must always be carried out if worthwhile changes are to be made in the staff development offerings. In other words, if one of the input factors is changed, evaluation must occur in order to determine the potential impact of the change on the other stages. If, for example, the agency redefined role expectations for nurse assistants, the expected outcomes would have to be evaluated in relation to the present input and process to determine what types of changes need to be made. Perhaps the new expectations would only require the addition of a small segment of content. On the other hand, they may alter the entire offering. Similarly, altering the design of the program has the potential to affect the total output. Without evaluation at this step, potential problem areas may be overlooked.

By definition, the evaluation is a *systematic approach* to establishing worth in terms of *predetermined standards*. The systematic approach requires that the collecting, organizing, analyzing, and reporting of information be accomplished before action is taken. The data are then measured against predetermined standards of accomplishment. These standards may emanate from the profession, an accrediting body, role expectations, goals, objectives, and policies. The standards in staff development include those for individual accomplishments as well as those for learning offerings and the total staff development effort. Individuals may be evaluated in terms of test results and performance behaviors, while the

total staff development effort or specific components may be evaluated in terms of the behavioral changes they effect. Because it is ongoing, evaluation of the learners occurs over a period of time and not at one specific point. Thus we may expect to observe performance behaviors at the end of a particular offering as well as some designated interval afterwards.

The purpose of evaluation is to acquire information to determine the effectiveness of the staff development process in achieving better nursing care. The information collected should either reaffirm the current situation or point to a need for redirection of efforts and activities.

GENERAL PRINCIPLES IN EVALUATION

Before launching into a discussion of some specifics in evaluation within staff development, we need to familiarize ourselves with some general evaluation principles. Table 10-1 gives the general principles as well as examples of their application within staff development.

As can be seen, it is vital to plan for evaluation whether of an individual or an offering. First, the budget must be able to support the evaluation activity since time and some materials are involved. The hypothetical learning offerings that follow exhibit the possible variance in time and materials.

1. The objective of this offering is stated as, "After viewing a film on diabetes, the learner will list four signs and symptoms of impending metabolic acidosis." The staff development educator could provide the learners with blank pieces of paper, allow time for them to write their responses, and then determine the correctness of the answers.

2. The objective of this offering is stated as, "After viewing a film on diabetes, the learner will list four signs and symptoms of impending metabolic acidosis, stating the causative factors for each." The staff development educator may wish to have the response forms divided into columns or sections for ease in reviewing the responses. Thus some secretarial time is involved. It will take longer for

Table 10-1. Evaluation principles

Principle	Application within staff development
Decisions about evaluation are an integral part of the planning phase of any learning offering.	The budget allows for evaluation of a learning offering. Evaluation is planned prior to conducting the learning offering.
Evaluation is stated in terms of performance behaviors.	Behavioral objectives are stated for each learning offering and serve as a basis for evaluation.
Evaluation criteria are clearly stated and define the parameters of behavior.	There is agreement on the meaning of terms for commonality in interpretation. The wording selected for a given classification of employees is in terms that the employees understand. The specified criteria give direction to the staff development educator in terms of the degree of competency an individual must demonstrate. More than one observation is made.
Evaluation statements specify the conditions under which the evaluation will occur.	The staff development educator knows where and when the evaluation occurs and what other, if any, conditions exist.
The scope of the evaluation process is predetermined.	Individuals as well as the staff development process are evaluated. The systematic approach specifies how the information will be collected, organized, analyzed, reported, and acted on. The process is continuous.
The evaluation process is shared with all those involved with it.	The learners know how they will be evaluated, the other staff know what is expected of them in terms of evaluation, and the staff development educator shares appropriate information. Evaluation is viewed as being more objective because everyone knows the criteria and receives feedback.
Feedback reinforces positive behaviors and redirects negative ones.	The staff development educator and others involved in evaluating learners keep the learners informed of their progress. In the evaluation of the staff development process, feedback from the staff gives direction to retaining certain approaches and content and reorganizing others.
Negative feedback is better than no feedback at all.	The staff development educator apprises the learners of negative behavior even if there is no positive behavior.

the staff development educator to review the responses because there is more information to be analyzed.

3. The objective of this offering is stated as, "After viewing a film on diabetes, the learner will assess diabetic patients, recording which signs and symptoms of impending metabolic acidosis are present (if any)." With this objective, it is necessary for the staff development educator to return to the clinical area with the learners in order to make the same observations they will make to determine if their responses are correct. Depending on the number of learners, the staff development educator

could be involved for some time in the clinical area.

4. The objective of this offering is stated as, "After viewing a film on diabetes, the learner will identify signs and symptoms of impending metabolic acidosis, correlating them with the causative factors." In this situation the staff development educator may need to prepare a variety of signs and symptoms and a list of potential causative factors. This pre-offering activity is time-consuming for the educator as well as for the secretary who will prepare the test for distribution. Some materials are used in preparing the necessary copies. The time required for reviewing results may be short if the grading is done electronically. (This approach may be expensive, however.)

In addition to budget considerations, planning for evaluation alerts all persons involved to expected activities and responsibilities. Many of us have been in situations where we have been handed an evaluation form to complete. Without advance preparation, we probably did not have the necessary facts or an understanding of the criteria. In other words, we were not able to make a fair, objective evaluation in the allotted time. Without some predetermination of what to expect from an offering or an individual, there are no criteria on which to base an evaluation.

Mager[2] cites three aspects of instructional objectives that we believe could be incorporated in evaluation. The three parts relate to (1) the behavior, (2) the criteria, and (3) the conditions. The second, third, and fourth principles in Table 10-1 relate to Mager's points. While it is not necessary to state the evaluation in terms of performance behaviors, when such expectations have been established, it certainly facilitates the evaluation. In Table 8-1 (p. 75) the behaviors appear in the third column of the format for a teaching plan. Although this may seem somewhat backward, these objectives are, in essence, the measurable outcomes of the learning offering. Thus one statement gives direction to planning content and teaching methods as well as providing the basis for evaluation.

The objective should guide both the learner and evaluator. An objective stated as, "Know the difference between left- and right-sided heart failure" is not explicit enough to give adequate direction to either the learner or evaluator. In the past such broadly stated objectives resulted in few problems because the learners really were not evaluated in terms of the objectives. In staff development we frequently did not make any evaluation even though we had stated objectives. However, if learning outcomes are going to be seriously evaluated, clearly defined guidelines must be established. In the previous example, if "know" were defined in terms of "list," "match," or "describe" a specific measuring device would be indicated.

Next, criteria of performance must be stated to define the parameters of behavior. Frequently a number of responses or observations are cited as the lower limit of acceptable performance. For example, in a nurse assistant orientation offering the learners might be required to turn patients every two hours. Thus even though the performance behavior (turning) may be present, it may not meet the criteria (every two hours).

In order for the learners to understand what is expected of them, the "language of the learner" must be used. For example, the directions a team leader might give to a new nurse assistant, "Observe the patient for untoward symptoms," are not so clear as, "Please note pedal edema." It would be even clearer to say, "Please tell me if you notice the feet swelling or getting puffy." Because words have different meanings for different people, it is desirable to know the potential interpretations before using certain words. If one word is particularly appropriate but confusing to those involved with its use, the standard interpretation could be given in a footnote. If many words are desirable but confusing, it may be necessary to attach a list of terms or additional delimiting terms. The important point to remember is that everyone, including the learners, must have the same understanding.

Additionally, evaluation statements denote the conditions under which evaluation will occur. In the example "Know the difference between left- and right-sided heart failure," the performance is not defined in terms of when (for example, immediately or two weeks after the completion of a course). Knowing when the performance is expected assists the staff development educator in planning for evaluation and the learners in knowing what is expected of them.

To determine the scope of the evaluation process, its various purposes must be viewed together. We have identified evaluation as it relates to both the learner and the staff development process. If behavioral objectives are established for the learner, it should not be difficult to ascertain whether or not the performance behavior is acceptable. In evaluating the staff development process, however, it will probably be necessary to expend more energy. First, each learning offering is evaluated in terms of whether or not the goals were met. As identified in Fig. 1-2, evaluation is incorporated at each and every step. Therefore the analysis of each step should occur as an offering is being developed, and it should occur at the end of the offering as a review analysis, especially if the resulting output did not include the desired performance behavior. Next, the total staff development effort is evaluated in terms of the overall goals. If each learning offering is successful, it is likely that the total effort will also succeed. Such may not be the case, however, if a learning offering essential to the attainment of a broad goal is omitted. Also, if evaluation is not incorporated throughout the staff development process, the changes in the input or process phases needed to achieve the desired output may not be effected.

The evaluation process also involves formulating value judgments. However, if the information has not been collected and organized in a systematic way, false conclusions may be reached. Most of us, for example, are aware of the "halo" effect, whereby the whole situation or person is evaluated in terms of only one aspect.

Inherent in evaluation is the concept of involving the necessary people in the process. If observations of the staff development educator are to be supplemented by those of other evaluators, these others must be prepared accordingly. Also, in order for an atmosphere of mutual trust to exist, the learners must know what is expected of them. If there has been a common understanding of the terms used and the behaviors expected, evaluation is viewed as more objective than if words and behaviors are not defined.

Finally, feedback is used to reinforce positive behavior and to redirect negative behavior. Without feedback, most people will assume that their behaviors and goals are acceptable. Similarly, when no feedback is received about a particular learning offering, it will probably be deemed acceptable even though it may be ineffective. Although positive reinforcement is always preferred, it should be remembered that a negative response is better than no response at all; while it does not instruct the individuals in desirable behavior, it does inform them that their present actions are unacceptable. Some individuals, however, may be frustrated by the negative feedback and decide to leave the situation. Thus, if positive behavior is expected, the individuals must know what is expected of them.

THE EVALUATION PROCESS WITHIN STAFF DEVELOPMENT

Before the evaluation process actually begins, the "who," "what," "when," "where," "how," and "why" factors must be considered. The "why" of evaluation has been identified already in the section on its purposes. The "who," "what," "when," and "where" were discussed in the previous section on application of the evaluation principles. "How" relates to the method to be used and was alluded to in the discussion of principles. "How" includes the techniques of evaluation that are described in the next section.

The evaluation process includes the following steps:

1. Collecting
2. Organizing
3. Analyzing
4. Reporting
5. Acting

The collection of data should proceed according to established criteria and some identified method. In staff development the goals for the total effort serve as its criteria. In a specific learning offering the objectives determine its criteria; the performance behaviors identify the learners' criteria. Thus one of the bases for collecting facts should be explicit from the development of learning offerings. The other aspect, the method of collection, deals with selecting the appropriate technique to obtain the desired information. Specific methods are discussed in the next section. The type of technique selected must be given careful consideration. One that is too complex will not be used by the personnel; one that is too simple will not provide the information needed.

In collecting data the potential sources must be determined. The learners are an obvious source. What they learned and how they perceive the learning experience is invaluable information regardless of whether the evaluation is aimed at the learners themselves, a specific offering, or the entire staff development process. If change in behavior has occured but the learners really disliked the approach used, the design of the learning offering should be reevaluated. If, on the other hand, the offering was enjoyable but did not produce the desired behavior, the content probably needs to be adjusted. The point is that the learners are a most valuable resource in the collection of data.

Other staff members, no doubt, have reactions to specific individuals or learning offerings. For instance, although the learners may have acquired the desired behavior, certain members of the staff may feel threatened because they did not become adequately involved in the experience. Thus implementing the desired change in behavior may produce interpersonal problems among the staff. Or, other staff members may find a change in the desired performance over a period of time and thus provide valuable input in terms of the lasting effects of staff development. The methods used in collecting such data vary with each case and one method should not be solely depended on.

Key persons in the agency can also provide some useful data. Perhaps the director of medical education has a contribution to make concerning medical-nursing programs; perhaps nursing administration can project future plans for nursing care; perhaps the social worker has some thoughts on how the staff uses a referral system. All these sources may be valuable. However, there should always be a specific reason for asking an individual to participate in any evaluation.

After collection, the data should be organized. Obviously it is desirable to know what end results are needed and how the information should be organized before a method of collection is developed. For instance, if statistical information in terms of agreement and disagreement is needed, a method should be used that forces a positive or negative response. It is amazing how many individuals are unable to respond directly to questions. Therefore if specific responses are desired, specific and pointed questions must be asked. Once received, it may be helpful to organize information by individual offerings, by the type of offering (clinical or employee classification), by individuals, or by some other predetermined means of differentiation.

After the data for an individual, an offering, or the total effort have been organized, they must be analyzed. Depending on the agency, analysis may involve refined statistical procedures or a simple categorization of the responses in terms such as "good," "bad," "achieved," or "failed." Whatever approach is used, the review of information should be consistent and involve a detailed analysis of the facts. This latter step is particularly crucial as it determines the significance of the evaluation facts. It is at this point that the "labels" of relative value appear.

Next, the findings must be reported. The report may be a tabulation of responses or a narrative description. In either case, it should be written for present documentation as well as future planning. When an individual is evaluated, he should be given a copy of his evaluation and at the very least be required to read and cosign it. In evaluating specific offerings, the evaluations should be summarized and attached to the file for that offering. In some cases the original facts (observations and responses) should be kept for future reference. Even after a learning offering has been altered it may be desirable to retain the original design and evaluation for future reference. In evaluating the total staff development effort, the "tone" of the evaluations should be incorporated in the annual report. It may be necessary to summarize the evaluation information for planning purposes.

Reports are presented to the various committees, administrators, clinical personnel, and related services as indicated by the results of the evaluation. The learners and their immediate supervisors obviously need to be involved, as does the director of the nursing service. Additionally, others may be involved, for instance, the librarian if the library resources were a topic of the evaluation.

The final step is action. The analysis of data should result in the formulation of conclusions. Thus there is a basis for acting—release the orientee to the service or retain the orientee until the learning needs are met; retain the current learning offering or revise it; continue with present endeavors or reevaluate their direction. Action should be initiated once convincing data have been obtained and not delayed while additional information is gathered, unless it will significantly alter the conclusions.

METHODS OF EVALUATION AND MEASUREMENT

The intent of this section is to provide a brief overview of some methods of evaluation and measurement that are useful in staff devel-

opment. There are numerous sources dealing specifically with evaluation and measurement that provide in-depth descriptions of the methods. Some of these sources appear in the bibliography.

The critical issue in determining the method to use is knowing what is to be evaluated. As already stated, the learners, the learning offering, and the total staff development effort must be evaluated. In the following discussion of some methods for evaluation, we have incorporated the three areas of evaluation within staff development to demonstrate how various techniques can be used to serve more than one end. Some methods are more suited for a particular type of information and thus may be very useful in one aspect of evaluation but less so in another. Again, evaluation is predetermined and incorporated into the staff development process. Evaluation is based on specific objectives, and these should guide the choice of an evaluation method.

Some of the following methods produce only quantitative results. They are incorporated in evaluation, however, to the extent that they produce certain data that are used to determine the worth of a response, individual, or situation. Whenever possible, it is advisable to incorporate more than one method in the evaluation process.

Anecdotal records

Webster's dictionary defines anecdote as a short, entertaining account of some happening, usually personal or biographical. In retrospect, some anecdotal records are entertaining even if they are not so designed. The anecdotal record describes the situation, what the learner did, and the evaluator's interpretation. Because there are no structured responses, there is greater opportunity to describe details. However, there is the potential hazard of jumping to conclusions rather than recording the facts. Considering that the anecdotal record includes the evaluator's interpretation, it is imperative that predetermined standards of performance are used so that the same situation is not described in a multitude of ways. While this method requires little advance preparation, the recording and analysis of information is somewhat time-consuming. In order to be representative of a learner's behavior, several anecdotal notations should be made. For convenience, a file box with alphabetical index cards might be used to store information about various individuals. Also, it may be advisable to indicate some specific categories of behavior to be observed.

The learners. Anecdotal notes for the individual are used to document demonstrated behavior in a simulated setting or in the clinical area. If individuals cannot perform in a simulated situation, they are not likely to be able to perform in the real situation. It should be remembered, however, that acceptable performance in a simulated situation does not necessarily indicate an ability to perform in the same manner in the real situation. These records are samples of typical behavior in relation to certain expected behaviors. A typical example might be as follows:

Individual's name

Date   **Assignment:** Team leader
    Febrile condition reported per nurse assistant for patient allergic to aspirin. Returned to patient's room, assessed physical status, and requested nurse assistant to secure two ice bags, recheck the temperature in 30 minutes, and report findings. Sought information when nurse assistant did not report within 45 minutes.
    • Recognizes appropriate action
    • Holds personnel accountable

In order for this behavior to be considered typical, similar incidents must be recorded. Some observers have a tendency to record only negative situations. While these are helpful in the overall effort, they represent only a segment of the whole situation.

The learning offering. Individuals' anecdotal records can be used to reflect the output from the learning offering. Because staff development seeks to change behavior through the teaching-learning process, the anecdotal records of the learners should show the effects of the learning offering.

Additionally, generalized anecdotal records noting the reactions of the learners to a particular offering might be helpful. Accumulation of such information gives direction to the future plans for the learning offering.

The staff development effort. An accumulation of anecdotal records for individuals and learning offerings provides information about the total effort. Usually a summary of the records rather than the original notations will suffice. However, it may be desirable to keep some specific records that are reflective of the observations made during the designated period.

Self-evaluation

The term "self-evaluation" implies that individuals evaluate their own situation or behavior and then relate it to expected outcomes. This approach usually requires another individual to observe at least portions of the situation or behavior in order to assist the learner in developing self-evaluation skills. For this method to have meaning for the individual, it is essential that a clear description of the expected output be available prior to evaluation. The data may be recorded in the form of a narrative or a list.

The learners. Self-evaluation for adult learners is especially beneficial because it allows them to express their own perceptions of a situation. They tend to develop a sense of responsibility for viewing their behavior in an objective way and for recording and reporting their findings. It is possible, however, that adults may be oriented to viewing a behavior or situation in a strictly defined way and thus may need assistance in broadening their viewpoints. Additionally, many learners may find this method somewhat threatening because they have had no previous exposure to it.

The learning offering. Self-evaluation within the learning offering may include the learners' perceptions of what they gained from a particular offering. It also implies that the staff development educator should analyze the learning offering in terms of the staff development process to determine the effectiveness of the offering.

The staff development effort. Again, an accumulation (or summary) of self-evaluations from the learners and staff development educators should give some direction to future planning.

Checklists

As the name suggests, a checklist is a listing, usually by category, of various expected outcomes. Some checklists indicate that the item is to be checked if observed; otherwise no notation is made. Others use a "yes" and "no" format. Sometimes other columns are added to indicate "not applicable" (NA) or "not observed" (NO).

The checklist takes time to prepare but is fairly easy to use because it forces responses in predetermined ways. Thus there is little potential for misunderstanding in the analysis phase. As with other methods, the checklist reports information in a given situation at a specific time. Therefore repeated use of checklists for evaluation is recommended.

The learners. One of the most common checklists is the "skills inventory" that many agencies use to determine the basic skills of new employees within a defined position. In this instance the responses are based on the individuals' perceptions of their abilities and not necessarily on present behavior. Thus it may be advisable for an independent observer to check whether or not the learners possess the skills they have identified. For instance, a checklist could be used in the clinical area by the head nurse to indicate what behaviors the learners have demonstrated. Also a checklist could be used at the termination of a learning offering for the learners to indicate their current abilities.

The learning offering. A checklist can be used by clinical personnel to indicate the behaviors that the learners did not demonstrate prior to participating in a specific offering. The checklists from the individuals can be summarized and used to estimate the value of the offering. Additionally, educators might de-

vise a checklist to determine if they have used the staff development process effectively.

The staff development effort. Within the total effort, checklists might be kept in terms of successful versus unsuccessful programs. The content of the checklist will relate to the steps in the staff development process. Some correlation between using the process and achieving desired results may be expected.

Rating scales

Rating scales are made up of descriptions of varying degrees of achievement. The terms used provide differentiation in the behavior or situation. These scales may be designed in columns to obtain the same kind of information for each aspect to be evaluated. Or the scales may be constructed to allow for different types of responses to each question.

The learners. A typical scale shows whether or not the learners have met the expectations. Therefore the usual categories are in such terms as "excels standard," "meets standards," and "does not meet standard." Numbers may also be used to represent these categories. There usually are three or five categories, with the middle one representing the average expectation. Unfortunately most rating scales are somewhat ambiguous, especially in their qualitative comparisons. Whenever possible, the behaviors that correspond to the terms used in the rating scale should be identified to standardize the interpretation of the terms.

The learning offering. Although changes in the behavior of learners is the most obvious indication of the effectiveness of an offering, a scale could be developed for the offering itself. The factors to be assessed in this scale usually relate to the content and the method of presentation. Typical rating terms are "most useful," "somewhat useful," "useful," and "not useful." Numbers may be used also. Information solicited from the learners should prove most helpful in evaluating the learning offering. In fact, if enough categories have been listed, the learners can help evaluate each factor in the staff development process. For example, a question about the time at which the offering was held or one about their perception of the learning needs can provide additional input in analyzing these steps in the process.

The staff development effort. In order to determine the effectiveness of the total staff development effort, a rating scale might be devised for use by select individuals. This scale should be broad enough to include all the types of offerings; for example, leadership development might be an appropriate category. The individuals selected to respond to this scale should be those who were involved with the learning situation and those who were involved with observing the changes in behavior (the persons in the clinical area to whom the learner is responsible). The resultant information should provide a basis for determining whether or not the overall goals were attained.

Tests

There are a variety of tests that can be used in staff development. Some of the more commonly used tests are described here. Generally they can be divided into two classifications—selected answers (objective) and self-constructed answers (essay). Within the category of objective tests, there are true-false multiple-choice, classification, and matching. Briefly, true-false tests are statements with which one must agree or disagree. Obviously there is a fifty-fifty chance of guessing the correct answer. This type of question can be tricky, however, when one part is obviously true and the other part is not so clearly true or false.

Multiple-choice tests provide a statement (the stem) followed by several options for completing it (the alternatives). Frequently the alternatives, which consist of the answer and distractors, are labeled. Sometimes one of the alternatives states "all of the above" or "none of the above." As with all tests, the multiple-choice test must be well constructed if it is to be effective.

Classification tests usually provide some basic information before presenting the questions. The responses to the questions are based on the prefacing information and take the

form of a classification of items, for example, the types of arrhythmias.

Matching tests involve comparing two groups of items and correlating them in some way. Frequently there is a condition or problem in one column that relates with one or more responses in another column. If there are an equal number of items in each column, the persons using the test may be able to guess those responses they do not really know.

While most tests measure quantity (number of correct responses), some can be designed to indicate quality, for instance, "indicate the *best* answer," in situations where there is more than one correct response.

An essay test allows individuals to express their understanding of a particular situation. A statement is made or a question is asked, and the learners are expected to respond accordingly. In order to be objective in reviewing responses, certain factors should be identified that are a necessary part of a correct response. These factors are compared with those included in the individuals' responses in order to assess the individuals' understanding of a situation.

The learners. Testing for the learners usually occurs at three points—pre, post, and follow-up. A pretest may be given to determine the present knowledge base, a post-test is administered to determine what change has resulted, and a follow-up test after some predetermined period can indicate retention of the information and consistency in the performance behavior.

The learning offering. The test results of the learners are frequently used to determine the effectiveness of a particular offering. It is conceivable that you may wish to design a test to determine the effectiveness of the offering. If this approach is used, the learners should be alerted, as they will need to familiarize themselves with process as well as the content.

The staff development effort. Generally, tests related to the total effort are not used. However, a test may be developed that relates to all offerings within a given period of time. There may be a wide range of responses due to the variation in attendance at all offerings. As with other methods, generalizations about the total effort can be made in light of learner progress and the demonstrated effectiveness of specific offerings.

Questionnaires, interviews, and surveys

As discussed in Chapter 7, information about learning needs can be gained by talking with others and by having them record certain information. If these same techniques are used subsequent to a learning offering, they can provide some information for evaluation purposes. For example, if all the supervisors indicate that the head nurses did not retain a specified behavior after a learning offering, there are implications for learning needs as well as for evaluation of the learning offering. Additionally, many agencies use patient surveys to determine the consumers' point of view.

Additional evaluation points

In addition to the previously discussed methods for analyzing change in behavior and effectiveness of the programming, it may be deemed necessary to review the participation of learners within the classroom setting. If it is decided that this is a significant factor, the pertinent observations should be recorded for future reference.

Attendance may be an important factor, also. If the learners are consistently late or absent, it is probably advisable to analyze the scheduling and other aspects of the learning offering. However, the individual's work attendance record should also be checked to determine if there is a consistent pattern of tardiness or absenteeism.

Review of incident reports may provide some indication of the effectiveness of programs dealing with safety. Certain types of incidents could be reviewed before and after a learning offering to determine if there has been a decrease in the frequency and severity of that particular type of incident.

The effectiveness of the method

No matter what method of evaluation is used, a few key points should be remembered

in providing feedback. Generally the greater the frequency of feedback, the greater the possibility of change in behavior, reinforcement of positive behaviors, and redirection of negative ones. If the learners do something incorrectly, they should be informed as quickly as possible so they can change their behavior. Comments should be specific so the learners understand the parameters of acceptable performance. Thus feedback will assist the learners to change their behavior in accordance with the expectations.

As stated previously, more than one observation or method should be used in evaluating a situation. An example of using a variety of methods appears in the Appendix (Exhibit P). Also, it should be remembered that the learners may be demonstrating compliance but not acceptance. That is, they conform to a behavior because they receive criticism when they do not; however, they do not really believe that the expected performance is desirable. It may be difficult to determine if compliance or acceptance is present in a specific situation. Thus repeated evaluations, especially by more than one individual, may provide some clues to the real basis for the behavior. We all know that there are individuals who perform in certain ways when certain others are present and immediately change their behavior when those individuals leave.

The selection of the method is determined by the kinds of information to be obtained, by the abilities of the staff development educators, and by the objectives of the offerings. No one method will produce consistently good results in all situations. Generally speaking, observation of change in behavior, especially over a period of time, is the most effective method for determining the worth of the staff development endeavors.

APPLICATION OF THE EVALUATION PROCESS

An initial step in evaluating the effectiveness of a program consists of reviewing a description of the program. The description should include the objectives, the content to be offered, the time required to meet the objectives, the target population, and all the learning resources to be utilized.

Each learning offering has one or more objectives that indicate the desired end results of the total effort. Each of these objectives may have a contributory or subobjective. Subobjectives must be attained before the overall objectives are reached. Most learning offerings will have subobjectives. All of the subobjectives are related in time to each other and to the total program objectives. A subobjective usually is stated specifically; that is, in planning it is decided whether they must be accomplished in order. In some offerings the first subobjective must be accomplished before the next one. The question becomes one of what is the real hierachy of learning; therefore it is usually necessary to rely on past experience or expert judgment. To illustrate, if the overall objective is to "give basic nursing care to the patient while under the supervision and direction of the registered nurse," there probably would be a number of subobjectives; for example, give a complete bed bath and give oral hygiene. The level of proficiency exhibited in one of the subobjectives may not influence the next one or assure a high level of success in attaining the overall objective.

The assumption may be made that each learning activity entailed in a subobjective will lead to the attainment of that particular objective, but that the attainment of all the subobjectives must be accomplished before the overall objectives can be attained. In evaluating the effectiveness of a learning offering, criteria of behavior or standards of accomplishment for each subobjective are applied. It is assumed that performing a planned learning activity will result in the attainment of the desired objectives. Again, there is a linkage between the subobjectives and the overall objectives as the behaviors become a set of performances versus one performance activity.

There is a range of acceptability in certain activities. To illustrate this, we can view a training program. In such a program, most of the output may be related to a "manual" type of performance and consequently the behav-

iors can be observed and more easily related to meeting performance requirements. The nature of an overall objective and the subobjectives are illustrated in this example. One overall objective of this learning offering states, "When assigned to provide basic nursing care to a patient on a nursing unit, the nurse assistant has the necessary manual and technical skills."

The learning offering has fourteen units. In units 4, 5, 6, 9, and 10 there are subobjectives of this overall objective. For example, unit 4 has a subobjective that states, "Can make an occupied or unoccupied bed for the patient." The content is bedmaking. The criteria of behavior for determining if the behaviors demonstrate attainment of the objective are stated as, "Demonstrates organization, neatness, manual dexterity, and conservation in efforts and use of linens." Observations of performance of the manual skills (a mitered corner, a smooth bed foundation) would be indicators for attainment. In unit 5 the subobjective states, "Utilizes principles of proper body mechanics in lifting, moving, positioning, ambulating and transporting patients or equipment." The criteria of behavior for determining the adequacy or completeness of the attainment of the stated subobjective would be (1) maintains proper body alignment and position of patient and of self when turning or moving the patient, when assisting patient to a sitting or dangling position, and when assisting or lifting patient onto cart or bed and placing patient in chair or returning to bed; (2) ambulates patient and can intervene appropriately to prevent injury if patient starts to fall; and (3) transports patient via cart or wheelchair, observing safety precautions. There is no limit to the number of subobjectives that may arise from the overall objectives.

IMPLICATIONS FOR EVALUATION

Information from any evaluation method can provide a basis for change and improvement or serve as a stimulus for future goal setting. Feedback indicating that the effectiveness of an offering is limited may lead to major changes in the offering. Or the feedback may show that the output is at the highest possible level, given the existing constraints or contingencies. One result of evaluation might be a change in the use of the resources, such as changing the ratio of instructors to participants or securing new hardware or software. One alternative may be to discontinue the learning offering. No amount of ingenuity in the evaluation process can eliminate the need to interpret the information and make the proper decision.

The evaluation process includes reviewing the philosophy and overall goals of staff development as progress is made toward long-range goals. Annual goals may result from the evaluation information. The need to review staff development efforts with line personnel must be planned and provided for to assist in evaluating the overall coordination and communication efforts.

Additionally, evaluation identifies strengths and weaknesses in the staff, the staff development educator, and the offerings. Without the evaluation information, the efforts may never meet the goals.

REFERENCES

1. Stufflebeam, D. L.: Toward a science of educational evaluation, Educ. Technol. 8:5, July, 1968.
2. Mager, R.: Preparing instructional objectives, Belmont, Calif., 1962, Fearon Publishers.

BIBLIOGRAPHY

Abedor, A. J., and Gustafson, K. L.: Evaluating instructional development programs: two sets of criteria, Audiovis. Instr. 16:21, Dec., 1971.

Aiken, L., and Aiken, J. L.: A systematic way to the evaluation of interpersonal relationships, Am. J. Nurs. 73:863, 1973.

Albrecht, S.: Reappraisal of conventional performance appraisal systems, J. Nurs. Admin. 1(2):29. 1972.

Bare, C. E.: Behavioral change through effective evaluation, J. Nurs. Educ. 6(4):7, 20, 1967.

Barrett, J.: The head nurse: her changing role, ed. 2, New York, 1968, Appleton-Century-Crofts.

Douglas, L. M., and Bevis, E. O.: Team leadership in action, St. Louis, 1970, The C. V. Mosby Co.

Drucker, P. F.: The practice of management, New York, 1954, Harper & Row, Publishers.

Gronlund, N. E.: Measurement and evaluation in teaching, New York, 1971, Macmillan Publishing Co., Inc.

Guinée, K. K.: The aims and methods of nursing education, New York, 1966, Macmillan Publishing Co., Inc.

Kimball, S. J., Pardee, G., and Larson, E.: Evaluation of staff performance, Am. J. Nurs. 71:1744, 1971.

Knowles, M. S.: The modern practice of adult education, New York, 1970, Association Press.

Litwack, L., Sakata, R., and Wykle, M.: Counseling, evaluation and student development in nursing education, Philadelphia, 1972, W. B. Saunders Co.

Mitsunaga, B. K.: Evaluation in continuing education, J. Nurs. Educ. 12(1):21, 1973.

National League for Nursing, Inc.: Evaluation—an objective approach, report of the 1971 workshops of the Council of Diploma Programs, New York, 1972, The League.

National League for Nursing, Inc.: Test construction and evaluation, workshop materials, New York, 1972, The League.

Nelson, C. H.: Measurement and evaluation in the classroom, London, 1970, Macmillan Publishing Co., Inc.

Palmer, M. E.: Self-evaluation of clinical performance, Nurs. Outlook 15:63, 1967.

Rines, A. R.: Evaluating student progress in learning the practice of nursing, New York, 1963, Teachers College Press.

Thompson, P. H., and Dalton, G. W.: Performance appraisal: managers beware, Harvard Bus. Rev. 48(1): 149, 1970.

Training and continuing education; a handbook for health care institutions, Chicago, 1970, Hospital Research and Educational Trust.

Training the supervisor, Personnel Methods Series No. 4, Washington, D. C., 1956, U. S. Government Printing Office.

Tyler, R. W.: Basic principles of curriculum and instruction, Chicago, 1949, University of Chicago Press.

Tyler, R. W., Gagne, R. M., and Scriven, M.: Perspectives of curriculum evaluation, Chicago, 1967, Rand McNally Co.

Waller, M. V., and Davids, D. J.: Performance profiles . . . based on nursing activities records, J. Nurs. Admin. 2(5):61, 1972.

Yura, H., and Walsh, M.: Guidelines for evaluation: who, what, when, where, and how? Supervisor Nurse 3(2): 33, 1972.

11 Future directions

The only thing constant is change.

ANONYMOUS

Change affects us daily in our personal as well as professional lives. The knowledge we were secure with yesterday may be totally outdated tomorrow. Never before have we felt less certain as to what the future will be like. How alert we are as staff development educators will affect how prepared we will be to meet future needs.

Today one of the chief responsibilities of any administrator, manager, or educator is to cope with change. We deal with change in our defined field as well as in related fields. For staff development educators this means that we must know, for example, what is happening in the health care field, education, psychology, labor relations, and sociology. Although our prime goal is to change the behavior of employees, we are affected greatly by the forces that bring about change. If we are prepared for potential change, we are more likely to deal with it in an organized manner than if we were not prepared. Planning for the future is like having "money for a rainy day"—it is there when needed.

CHANGES IN HEALTH CARE DELIVERY

How health care is delivered will influence us greatly. For example, the concepts of primary care and prevention imply that we approach patient care with a different orientation. Never before has so much emphasis been placed on patient education, an integral part of both concepts. Generally speaking, nursing has not made its primary focus on the well client or the one who has become ill but requires only a minimum of care. Community health nurses have devoted their time to the well and self-care clients, but some efforts have been severely restricted by limited funds and staff. As more efforts are made in prevention and primary care, the patient population in hospitals will change: the percentage of acutely ill patients will increase. With the advent of extended care facilities, patients may be exposed to more than one type of institutional care during a period of illness.

As agencies become more specialized, patients may be separated geographically from their families during illnesses requiring intensive care. Many people from rural or sparsely populated areas may have to go to nearby major cities to obtain intensive care. As a result, the family members may need help in order to cope with the situation. The geographical gap may pose difficulties for the family in preparing for the return of the family member. Thus, in addition to the change in patient population, the need for a communications system becomes crucial. Therefore two areas of concern for staff development educators are (1) the focus of future programming on the anticipated patient population and (2) exploration of communications systems for use within the agency and between agencies.

Coupled with a change in the delivery system is the issue of national health insurance. Although there is great controversy about how such a program should be developed, there is general consensus that it is inevitable. Some groups wish to have this insurance program developed along the lines of Medicare and Medicaid. Others demand a revision of the health care system to prevent additional wasted monies in an "antiquated" (as they view it) system. Some people advocate a "free for all" basis, while others seek a plan based on need. No matter what plan emerges, it will definitely affect the health care field to the extent that changes will result within most agencies. It behooves us as staff development educators to be alert to all national legislation dealing with health care.

IMPACT OF TECHNOLOGY

The time gap between the development of scientific theories and their practical application is decreasing. Technology is moving so rapidly that it is difficult to keep pace with it. More research is conducted, resulting in more reports and recommendations. Whether the advances occur within the health care field or within education, they have the potential to affect us. Technology within health care influences the content of staff development, whereas technology within education influences its methodology.

New pieces of equipment or modifications of present items are appearing constantly. There is the potential for an almost constant product turnover that may or may not cause greater involvement with reorientation. The educational resources in nursing have been modified greatly in the past few years. Considering all the fields with which staff development educators should be familiar, it is no wonder that we feel as if we are running to stay behind. For example, increase in the number of nursing journals alone has significantly affected the time devoted to reading.

Advances in automation have facilitated the handling of masses of information, reduced time in collection and correlation of information, and organized information into appropriate segments. Automation makes yesterday's discoveries available to more people much more rapidly. The staff development educator must be aware of technological advances in order to plan for the future even in a setting where automation is not much in evidence, for it well may be in the near future. For example, the use of computers has increased in hospital settings. They are being used in greater number and for a wider range of functions. In the future there will likely be computer-assisted practice, just as currently there is computer-assisted instruction. We will be able to retrieve nursing care information about patients just as easily as we retrieve instructional information.

Hardware and software may also be expected to change. More administrators recognize the advantages to staff development efforts within the agency and thus more adjuncts are being sought. If an agency does not possess a particular piece of equipment or learning system, it is possible that it will be available on loan from a nearby agency.

RESEARCH

In the nursing profession as well as in the total health care field, research will have new impact. Clinical nursing research will provide documentation of rationale for decision making and will be more quickly translated into practice. In addition, more agencies will begin to conduct their own research. Also, more research will be available to staff development educators as they develop new approaches. In addition to the clinical research, staff development educators will have more information about the teaching-learning process, climate setting, the effects of education and experience on the individual learner, and predictions of new graduates' clinical performance.

HEALTH TEAM APPROACH

As new groups emerge within the health field and as various existing groups alter their roles, more interdependence will result. For example, registered nurses are identifying their independent functions in such a way as to clarify for others that they do not work under someone's specific direction and that they are personally accountable to the public for their acts. Physicians continue to specialize in a given aspect of medicine and to define the needs for certain additional skills. Hospitals are seeking dietitians and social workers to deal with specific problems. Physical therapists and occupational therapists are brought to patient conferences to broaden the focus on patient problems.

We find articles and speeches advocating the elimination of the "pyramid" concept of the health team (with the physician at the top) and emphasizing the "pie" concept (with all members of the team interdependent). How staff development educators relate within the pie setting differs from how they relate within the pyramid setting. This change in focus no longer makes one person, or type of person, accountable for all decisions affecting the patients' care. Thus staff development educators need to be alert to who is responsible for what. Even within the field of nursing, the pyramid concept is undergoing change. Many agencies use a decentralized administrative approach, so that head nurses (or whatever the nurses responsible for given units are called) have more responsibility for controlling their own units. In some settings, policies are made at the unit level and concurrence is sought from the other areas affected by the decision. This approach differs considerably from that of policies emanating from the nursing administration office with impact on all clinical services. Again, the staff development educator needs to be alert to the changing roles and responsibilities within nursing.

CHANGING ROLES OF THE NURSING TEAM MEMBERS

In addition to the changes that affect the administration of nursing or the concepts of the health team, there are changes within nursing practice itself that alter the role of the registered nurse. For example, nurses traditionally have been data collectors. Now they are data interpreters as well. In the future we will see more interpretations being made by nurses and more nursing diagnoses being formulated. Nurses, being accountable to the consumers of health care, will assume different kinds of responsibilities in providing nurs-

ing care, including the involvement of clients and their families in formulating goals. They will develop plans that are suitable for the recipients of the care and will document these plans. Their decisions about nursing care, as reflected in nursing orders, may have legal significance as do a physician's orders for medical care. Nurses will be extending their roles as well as expanding their traditional roles in nursing practice. Obviously the nursing care approaches with which the staff development educator needs to be familiar will differ from those commonly in use today.

Legal aspects will become more crucial to nursing practitioners. For example, the significance of nursing orders needs to be understood before new directions are undertaken. Keeping abreast of legal changes becomes a critical responsibility for staff development educators.

Other members of the nursing team will face role changes also. Because of increased technology, licensed practical nurses will be expected to know more about the various measures taken in patient care. Nurse assistants will be used in differing ways, also, because of the increased patient demand for complex, highly skilled care. Other members of the nursing team with more well-defined parameters may not be affected too greatly. For example, the operating room technicians, while facing change, probably will not have a major role reversal.

Essential to the changing roles of registered nurses is the change in preparatory programs. Many baccalaureate programs are focusing on primary care. Baccalaureate graduates of such programs will be more highly skilled in client assessment and will be able to develop care plans that differ from those currently in existence. Thus we may anticipate a very different product within nursing services. Concurrently, many hospital-based programs have reduced the period of study to two academic or calendar years. Thus the new diploma graduates may not be so highly skilled as they have been in the past because of the decreased amount of time for clinical practice. Next, some of the associate degree programs have incorporated leadership as a content area within the basic program. Graduates of these programs may function in new ways.

The preparatory programs for licensed practical nurses have undergone some changes too. Much of the content has become more sophisticated and the new product differs from that previously developed.

While it is not the staff development educator's prime responsibility to know the basic educational programs, it is essential to know in general the content and basic differences. If the agency generally employs most of its nurses from specific programs, the faculty of these programs might be consulted as to the directions planned for the next several years. When such information is received in advance, there should be adequate time to plan for changing roles of current employees, create new positions, or develop orientation programs to meet the anticipated needs.

Finally, there are numerous basic "aide training courses" and many applicants for nurse assistant positions have completed such a course prior to coming to the agency. Although many courses follow a standard format, it will be necessary for the staff development educator and the new employer to scrutinize the previous learning experience for several years to come.

In adition to the directions many programs are taking, some are incorporating a work-study approach. Thus we may find some registered nurses who are seeking advanced academic preparation planning their schedules around their class time. Similarly, licensed practical nurses may be enrolled in a course to prepare them to become registered nurses, and nurse assistants may enroll in licensed practical nurse programs. Staff development educators need to be aware of such situations for various reasons. It may explain why specific individuals never attend continuing education offerings. It also may explain why certain employees begin to change their behavior. The staff development educator as a counselor should be aware of the programs that offer the work-study approach in the event a nursing employee expresses a desire to pursue formal education.

CAREER ORIENTATION

Although there is controversy surrounding career ladders and lattices, most educators agree that there should be some way to recognize past learning and to accelerate the new. No matter how it develops in specified settings, the concept of allowing for individual differences in pursuing a curriculum should be accepted. Thus the employee may frequently be away from the work setting in order to pursue additional educational opportunities in a formal setting. Although it is hoped that the new role will result in new behaviors, this does not always happen. Staff development educators need to be alert to the role conflict that some persons may face. Helping people to assume different roles becomes increasingly important.

EMPLOYEE BENEFITS

In future as in recent years, employees will seek improved benefits such as longer vacations (or other days off) and shorter working hours. If given more free time, some employees might seek educational opportunities. Some bargaining groups have already incorporated some kind of educational offering into employment contracts. While some groups will seek "on-the-job training," others will pursue some kind of monetary allowance for individuals wishing to attend programs outside the agency. Staff development educators therefore have a responsibility to be aware of outside offerings. Additionally, they may be responsible for making appropriate recommendations to various individuals.

PEER REVIEW

Peer review allows for a group of nursing colleagues to evaluate performance. Before the nurses meet, criteria for evaluation are established. These criteria are then applied to a given nursing care situation. In the course of the analysis, certain sanctions are indicated and practitioners are held accountable for their acts. Information can be derived from peer review situations that may indicate some learning needs. Peer review may be used before and after the introduction of a variable such as a new assessment program to determine the change that may be attributable to it. Staff development educators will need to be familiar with the process to assist others in conducting peer review as well as in evaluating their own performances.

VOLUNTARY OR MANDATORY CONTINUING EDUCATION

The profession is faced with the question of how it will maintain competency, and one of the avenues most likely to be considered will be continuing education. If continuing education is so critical to continued competency, we will need to examine carefully the best approach and its impact on practice.

At the 1971 American Nurses' Association Convention, one of the meetings on continuing education focused on what a few selected states were doing. One of the state representatives pointed out that legislation making something mandatory does not always do what it is intended to do. People cannot be forced to learn; presence of body does not necessarily mean presence of mind. Without the demonstrable behavior, it is difficult to know if someone has learned or not.

On the other hand, national statistics demonstrate that many nurses are not continuing learners.[1] They have failed voluntarily to demonstrate individual accountability for maintaining competence in their practice through continuing education efforts.

Evaluation will determine the relationship between continuing education and clinical competency. What the learners know when they enter a learning situation must be determined. In some instances a planned program may not be useful to certain learners because they will already be familiar with the content. Therefore it would not be advantageous to have them attend the program. They may, however, have difficulty applying their knowledge and need assistance in this area. In the future it will be more acceptable to have

"library time" and to allow individuals to attend portions of programs based on their documentated learning needs. We will be more likely to do this because there will be more in the literature dealing with the identification of learning needs of adults.

We will need to be more alert to the factors that prevent nurses from applying their new knowledge. "We've always done it that way" seems to be a favorite answer that we have tended to use at one time or another. Economics, staffing patterns, physician influence, and the physical setting all influence how readily a nurse can implement a new idea. Yet we see situations where nurses are condemned because "money was spent to train them, but there is no difference in performance." Because of the increased demands on the health care system and its funds, the effects of continuing education and staff development must be documented in terms of consumer benefits and personnel benefits.

Compliance with a voluntary system is one big problem; enforcement of a mandatory system in terms of improved clinical competence is another. We will need to look closely at continuing education efforts in terms of its effects on clinical practice, its geographical feasibility for the practitioners, and its acceptance by the profession.

Two significant aspects of this issue are the individual's responsibility and the financing of continuing education. As defined in Chapter 1, continuing education requires active participation on the part of the learner. If individuals do not assume responsibility for learning, they will not learn. The educator, however, must be cognizant of certain handicaps to learning—the offering is not geographically realistic, the offering does not meet the need, there is little opportunity to implement the new knowledge, the offering is economically unrealistic, or the climate prevents the implementation of the idea. The individual must be involved in the decision to attend a specific program or there may be no "return" commitment. The agency by reimbursing the individual in some way (paid time off, paid expenses, paid fees) has a concomitant responsibility to permit that individual to return with new knowledge that can be applied or tested within the agency when it is appropriate to the setting. We may expect that the agency's use of educational monies, including that for outside efforts, will be scrutinized.

Another facet of financing continuing education is particularly significant for individuals who will be paying their own expenses. All agencies that expect a fee for an offering must look realistically at what the fee includes and whether it is a reasonable amount to expect the group of learners to pay. This will be particularly important if we develop mandatory continuing education as one criterion for renewal of licensure. We will need to be particularly alert to the sponsor of the program, its objectives, the expectations and cost, and its acceptability within the context of the established criteria.

Even if continuing education is not made a requirement for relicensure, some agencies will have their own mandatory requirements. For example, some agencies may require a given number of contact hours or continuing education units (CEU) for continued employment. Others may require completion of cer-

tain courses for designated positions, for example, a leadership program prior to assuming a head nurse position.

As mandatory requirements within the agency develop, we must examine our systems of records and rewards. First, records must include the information necessary to document an individual's continuing education efforts. One of the recent attempts at standardization is the development of the CEU.[2] Basically, one CEU represents ten contact hours in a planned continuing education effort. There must be responsible sponsorship, adequate direction, and qualified instruction. If the agency decides to use the CEU, it must assume responsibility for maintaining the records. The National Task Force on the Continuing Education Unit identifies thirteen points to be recorded, eight of which are necessary for a sound record-keeping system. In addition to the name of the individual learner, the social security number should be recorded. The title of the program and a brief description as well as time, location, and format are designated. The number of CEU's is noted on this record to document the number of actual contact hours for the individual. An abbreviated example of a record for CEU's follows:

Individual attendance record

19 _____

_____   Standard for agency _____
Name   Last   First

_____   Number accumulated _____
          Social security No.

DATE   TITLE OF PROGRAM*   LOCATION†   CEU

*Describe program briefly (e.g., objectives) and designate format used.
†If outside of agency, indicate sponsor.

INSTITUTIONAL LICENSURE

Credentialing through an employer as opposed to having individual licensure is a critical issue. Some of the bases for recognition as a profession are a special education, accountability to the public, and standard expectations. Professional organizations have supported individual licensure as one way of remaining accountable to the public. If individual licensure were relinquished in favor of institutional licensure, laws that define the preparation and expectation of a type of practitioner would be eliminated. Rather, as is proposed, the employing agencies would completely control the qualifications and practice of all health workers except physicians. The agency would assume greater responsibility for meeting the educational needs because persons could assume a variety of different roles. Individuals, however, might have difficulty moving from one institution to another since each could establish its own criteria and evaluation system. In addition to confusing the practitioner, the public could be confused also. The premise of institutional licensure is that each individual would be evaluated in terms of abilities and potentials and then assigned to a certain position. The agency might have certain preservice educational requirements as well as educational criteria to be met within the agency. Thus all health care practitioners except physicians could possibly undergo changes in their preparation as well as role.

DEPARTMENTS OF EDUCATION WITHIN THE AGENCY

Staff development educators need to be alert to changes within the organizational structures of agencies. More agencies will examine the need for an agency-wide department to meet the learning needs of all employees. Generally, this department would be headed by an expert, perhaps with a doctorate in education. This individual would be responsible for all agency-wide offerings. In some settings the nursing staff development educators would be under this department, but the nursing department would still be responsible for identifying the learning needs of its practitioners. In order to use this approach, it is imperative to have qualified people in the nursing department who are able to identify needs and to evaluate clinical performances. In other settings the nursing staff development educators will remain under the nursing department. They will, however, work in liaison with the personnel in the agency-wide department to identify common learning needs of all employees in order to avoid duplication of efforts.

It is crucial that staff development educators be alert to various organizational patterns and know what potential problems and benefits exist with each. The organization of the agency and the philosophy of staff development will directly affect the role and position of the educator within that agency. In order to know if an agency will meet your expectations, you will need to examine its organization and philosophy in comparison with the expectations you have for implementing staff development.

SUMMARY

Briefly, we have discussed a few of the critical issues facing staff development educators. Omission of some particular aspect does not necessarily mean that we view it as insignificant. Rather, we hope this chapter will provide a few clues for additional study as well as stimulate interest in examining developments that affect staff development.

REFERENCES
1. Western Interstate Commission for Higher Education: Continuing education in nursing, Boulder, Colo., 1969, The Commission.
2. National Task Force on the Continuing Education Unit: The continuing education unit, Raleigh, N. C., 1970, The Task Force.

BIBLIOGRAPHY
Abdellah, F. G., et al.: New directions in patient-centered nursing: guidelines for systems of service, education and research, New York, 1973, Macmillan Publishing Co., Inc.
American Nurses' Association: An interim statement on continuing education in nursing, Kansas City, Mo., 1972, The Association.

Ayers, R., and Mayers, M. E.: Anatomy of a model practice act, J. Nurs. Admin. 2(1):34, 1972.

Barker, M.: The era of the computer and its impact on nursing, Supervisor Nurse 2(8):26, 1971.

Bates, B.: Doctor and nurse: changing roles and relations, N. Engl. J. Med. 283:129, 1970.

Bennis, W. G., et al.: The planning of change, ed. 2, New York, 1969, Holt, Rinehart & Winston, Inc.

Boehm, G. A. W.: Futurism: not oracles, planners. They're working to shape tomorrow, Think 36:16, July-Aug., 1970.

Boyle, R. E.: Articulation: from associate degree through master's, Nurs. Outlook 20:670, 1972.

Brown, E. L.: Nursing reconsidered, a study of change. I. The professional role in institutional nursing, Philadelphia, 1970, J. B. Lippincott Co.

Brown, E. L.: Nursing reconsidered, a study of change. II. The professional role in community nursing, Philadelphia, 1971, J. B. Lippincott Co.

Bullough, B.: The new militancy in nursing, Nurs. Forum 10:273, 1971.

Bullough, B., and Bullough, V.: A career ladder in nursing: problems and prospects, Am. J. Nurs. 71:1939, 1971.

Burnside, I. M.: Peer supervision: a method of teaching, J. Nurs. Educ. 10(4):15, 1971.

Chapman, J. K.: Annual administrative reviews: education, Hospitals 45(7):53, 1971.

Cleland, V., and Zagornik, D.: Appropriate utilization of health professionals, J. Nurs. Admin. 1(6):37, 1971.

Connors, E. J.: Annual administrative reviews: delivering and financing of health care, Hospitals 46(7):71, 1972.

Cooper, S. S., and Allison, E. W.: Should continuing education be mandatory? Am. J. Nurs. 73:442, 1973.

Cooper, S. S., and Hornback, M.: Continuing nursing education, New York, 1973, McGraw-Hill Book Co.

Extending the scope of nursing practice, Am. J. Nurs. 71:2346, 1971.

Farlee, C., et al.: A role for nurses in implementing computerized hospital information systems, Nurs. Forum 10:330, 1971.

Gibbs, G.: Will continuing education be required for license renewal? Am. J. Nurs. 71:2175, 1971.

Goldstein, B.: Characteristics of nursing units and accommodation to technological change, Nurs. Res. 21(1):63, 1972.

Gordon, T. J., and LeBleu, R. G.: Employee benefits, 1970-1985, Harvard Bus. Rev. 48(1):93, 1970.

Goshen, C. E.: Your automated future, Am. J. Nurs. 72:62, 1972.

Grand, N. K.: Nightingalism, employeeism, and professional collectivism, Nurs. Forum 10:289, 1971.

Hepner, J. O., and Hepner, D. M.: The health strategy game: a challenge for reorganization and management, St. Louis, 1973, The C. V. Mosby Co.

Ingles, T.: Debate: ladder concept in nursing education. Pro . . . , Nurs. Outlook 19:726, 1971.

Kisch, A. I.: Planning for a sensible health care system, Nurs. Outlook 20:640, 1972.

Kolodruhetz, W. W.: Two decades of employee-benefits plans, Soc. Sec. Bull. 35:10, April, 1972.

Kramer, M.: Team nursing—a means or an end? Nurs. Outlook 19:648, 1971.

Kriegel, J.: People are not resistant to change, Supervisor Nurse 2(11):35, 1971.

Laird, O. M.: Medical records, Hospitals 40(7):109, 1966.

Leininger, M.: This I believe—about interdisciplinary health education for the future, Nurs. Outlook 19:787, 1971.

Levey, S., and Loombs, N. P.: Health care administration: a managerial perspective, Philadelphia, 1973, J. B. Lippincott Co.

Lewis, C. E.: Annual administrative reviews: health manpower, Hospitals 46(7):107, 1972.

Licensure of health occupations, J.A.M.A. 208:2154, 1969.

Lorig, K.: Training health careerists in a service setting, J. Nurs. Admin. 2(1):59, 1972.

McGriff, E. P.: A case for mandatory continuing education in nursing, Nurs. Outlook 20:712, 1972.

MacPhail, J.: An experiment in nursing: planning, implementing and assessing planned change, Cleveland, 1972, Francis Payne Bolton School of Nursing.

Mason, E. J., and Barascandola, J.: Preparing tomorrow's health care team, Nurs. Outlook 20:728, 1972.

Montag, M.: Debate: ladder concept in nursing education. Con . . . , Nurs. Outlook 19:727, 1971.

Moore, A. J.: The ladder and the lattice, Nurs. Outlook 20:330, 1972.

National Commission for the Study of Nursing and Nursing education: An abstract for action, New York, 1970, McGraw-Hill Book Co.

National Commission for the Study of Nursing and Nursing Education: Continuing education in nursing: necessity and opportunity, Rochester, N. Y., The Commission.

National League for Nursing, Inc., Council of Baccalaureate and Higher Degree Programs: Challenge to nursing education—preparation of the professional nurse for future roles, Pub. No. 15-1420, New York, 1971, The League.

National League for Nursing, Inc., Council of Baccalaureate and Higher Degree Programs: Challenge to nursing education—professional nursing practice, New York, 1972, The League.

National League for Nursing, Inc., Council of Baccalaureate and Higher Degree Programs: Current issues in nursing education; papers presented, Pub. No. 15-1473, New York, 1972, The League.

Richardson, F. M.: Peer review of medical care, Med. Care 10:29, Jan.-Feb., 1972.

Rubin, C. F., et al.: Nursing audit—nurses evaluating nursing, Am. J. Nurs. 72:916, 1972.

Sanazaro, P. J., and Slosberg, B.: Annual administrative reviews: patient care evaluation, Hospitals 45(7):131, 1971.

Schlesinger, D. A.: Administrative reviews: health education, Hospitals **47**(7):137, 1973.

Schlotfeldt, R. M.: This I believe—nursing is health care, Nurs. Outlook **20**:243, 1972.

Shetland, M. L.: An approach to role expansion—the elaborate network, Am. J. Public Health **61**:1959, 1971.

Skarupa, J. A.: Management by objectives: a systematic way to manage change, J. Nurs. Admin. **1**(2):52, 1971.

Somers, A. R.: Health care delivery—university hospital: future role, J. Nurs. Admin. **2**(3):39, 1972.

Somers, A. R.: Health care in transition: directions for the future, Chicago, 1971, Hospital Research & Educational Trust.

Startsman, T. S., et al.: The attitudes of medical and paramedical personnel toward computers, Comput. Biomed. Res. **5**:218, 1972.

Stimpert, W.: Annual administrative reviews: education, Hospitals **47**(3):121, 1973.

Toffler, A.: Future shock, New York, 1970, Random House, Inc.

Tomasovic, E. R.: Turning nurses on to automation, Hospitals **46**(9):80, 1972.

Training and continuing education; a handbook for health care institutions, Chicago, 1970, Hospital Research & Educational Trust.

U. S. Department of Health, Education, and Welfare, Office of Assistant Secretary for Health: Report on licensure and related health personnel credentialing, DHEW Pub. No. (HSM) a72-11, Washington, D. C., 1971, U. S. Government Printing Office.

Yaw, R. D.: Annual administrative reviews: health care delivery, Hospitals **45**(7):87, 1971.

APPENDIX

Exhibit A

STAFF DEVELOPMENT POLICIES*

PREAMBLE

The Department of Nursing recognizes its responsibility for providing learning opportunities and an exemplary learning climate that will assist staff in becoming increasingly knowledgeable and competent in fulfilling role expectations. In turn, it expects the employees to identify and seek opportunities for learning based on their individual needs.

Staff development has two main compo-

nents, orientation and continuing education. Skill training and leadership development are integral parts of both. Participation in professional and related community activities is also viewed as contributing to the continued development of staff.

The focus in programming is on the knowledge, understanding, and skill required for nursing staff to increase their competencies in providing nursing care to patients. Formal as well as informal learning opportunities are utilized in both centralized and decentralized programs.

*Courtesy University Hospitals of Cleveland, Cleveland, Ohio; from Nursing Organization Manual, Feb., 1972.

POLICIES

Orientation

| PROGRAM | PART I | PART II | |
	INITIAL ORIENTATION	BASIC LEADERSHIP DEVELOPMENT	FOLLOW-UP CONFERENCE
Participants	RN's, LPN's, NTA's, NA's division secretaries	RN's	LPN's, NTA's, division secretaries
Attendance	Required, but exceptions may be made by assistant director based on: a. Role expectations for clinical service b. Individual employee's learning needs	Required before participation in promotional leadership development workshops	Required before participation in promotional conferences
Compensation	Considered to be "on-duty" time for payroll purposes; refer to *Administrative Policies and Procedures*	Same	Same

Continuing education

PROGRAM	PROMOTIONAL	MEDICATION COURSE	OTHER REQUIRED PROGRAMS
Participants	RN's, LPN's, NTA's, division secretaries	LPN's	As indicated by role and function
Attendance	Required before promotion to new position	Required for LPN's assigned to med-surg, ob-gyn, and psychiatric service except HP 2; exceptions made by staff development instructor if LPN satisfactorily demon-strates knowledge and skill in safe ad-ministration of drugs	Based on changing needs in nursing practice and/or role expectations
Compensation	Considered to be "on-duty" time for payroll purposes; refer to *Adminis-trative Policies and Procedures*	Same	Same

Continuing education

PROGRAM	VOLUNTARY PROGRAMS	PROFESSIONAL AND COMMUNITY ORGANIZATION ACTIVITIES
Participants	As indicated by role and function	All nursing personnel
Attendance	Based on individual needs and desires	Voluntary—personnel encouraged to accept nominations for offices as delegates or appointments to committees in professional and community organizations; before acceptance, provision made with director or her designee to be released to attend if elected or appointed; preference for attendance at activities given to officers, delegates, committee members, and other members.
Compensation	Compensation for payroll purposes not given if individual attends when scheduled to be off duty and is not expected or requested to attend program as part of his role/position*	Refer to *Administrative Policies and Procedures*

*Revision approved by Nursing Advisory Council, Sept. 14, 1972.

Exhibit B

PHILOSOPHY OF STAFF DEVELOPMENT*

The philosophy of staff development is based on the philosophy of nursing that identifies its obligation to society as the continuous "search for means to improve nursing practice and the delivery of health care."

Quality nursing care is dependent on the individual and collective abilities of the persons offering this care in relation to the needs of persons served and their readiness to accept and utilize services offered. Role expectations delineated for various categories of nursing personnel are based on differences in educational preparation, continued learning, and experience. The main purpose of staff development is to assist staff in becoming increasingly knowledgeable and competent in fulfilling role expectations.

Identifying and seeking learning opportunities are perceived as responsibilities of both the individual and the hospital. Joint efforts are evidenced by the establishment of an exemplary learning climate in which clinically competent role models play an important part in providing opportunities for learning. Although all involved in nursing practice serve as role models for others, certain persons are viewed as primary role models. These include senior clinical nurses, nurse clinicians, directors and assistant directors, and staff development instructors. Faculty of the Case Western Reserve University School of Nursing are viewed as an important part of the learning environment for nursing staff just as the staff

*Courtesy University Hospitals of Cleveland, Cleveland, Ohio; from Nursing Organization Manual, May, 1971 (approved by Nursing Council, Jan., 1971).

are considered as an important part of the learning climate for students. Assistant directors and senior clinical nurses are responsible within each clinical area for identification of learning needs, provision of opportunities for meeting these needs, and integration and evaluation of all learning activities in which their staff members are involved.

It is believed that staff development has two main components, orientation and continuing education. Skill training and leadership development are integral parts of both components.

Orientation is the introduction of the individual into a new situation. Some aspects are of immediate concern, while others of greater complexity are more effectively introduced at a later time. It is expected that the profile and goals of the individual and the basic role expectations will be used as a guide for planning and developing orientation.

Continuing education includes formal as well as informal learning opportunities planned for nursing staff following the basic orientation period. Provision is made for utilization of centralized as well as decentralized staff development programs. Some programs are centralized for purpose of efficiency and economy of operation, such as the skill training program for NTA's and the medication program for LPN's. Other programs are decentralized because they focus on knowledge, understanding, and skill required of nursing staff to care for specific patient populations. Most continuing education opportunities are planned on a decentralized basis.

Participation in professional and related

community activities is also viewed as contributing to the continued development of staff.

Workshops and individual guidance are methods used to develop leadership potential of registered nurses who are prepared through education for beginning leadership. Attention is devoted to problems of nursing practice, to directing and developing personnel involved in nursing practice, to providing continued learning opportunities for self and others, and to increasing potential in clinical competence.

It is believed that the goals of "improving nursing practice and the delivery of health care," and increasing opportunities for staff satisfaction can be facilitated by meeting the learning needs of nursing personnel. These goals will only be accomplished, however, if the individual utilizes the varied learning opportunities made available to him.

Exhibit C

CENTRALIZED STAFF DEVELOPMENT*

Purpose

The primary purpose of staff development is to assist staff in becoming increasingly knowledgeable and competent in fulfilling role expectations.

Goals

1. Provide a climate that fosters learning and thereby assists employees in adapting to their role within the hospital environment.
2. Assist individuals in identifying own learning needs.
3. Identify learning needs of groups of personnel.
4. Collaborate with clinical nursing personnel in determining learning needs of individuals and groups.
5. Plan, implement, and evaluate learning opportunities designed to assist the employees in fulfilling their role expectations.
6. Provide opportunities for continued learning that will assist the employees to develop to their potential in providing care for a specific patient population.
7. Provide audiovisual resources and consultation that will enhance learning opportunities for centralized and decentralized programs.
8. Assist clinical personnel with decentralized staff development by direct participation in planning and implementation of learning opportunities and by serving as a consultant and a role model.
9. Facilitate a constructive working relationship with clinical personnel and faculty of the School of Nursing in planning, implementing, and evaluating the centralized staff development program.
10. Utilize the unique contributions of members of other health disciplines in providing learning opportunities.

*Courtesy University Hospitals of Cleveland, Cleveland, Ohio.

Exhibit D

DECENTRALIZED STAFF DEVELOPMENT: MATERNITY AND GYNECOLOGY SERVICE*

Philosophy

The entire staff development program is organized around the concept that nursing care must consistently be based on standards, that these standards must reflect high expectations of care, and that these must be instilled in all nursing personnel expected to carry them out. The care standards are determined by the nursing personnel responsible for care in a given area, for example, senior clinical nurse, nurse clinician, supervisors, assistant director, director, and other nursing personnel. The role of the person responsible for staff development is to assist in instilling these standards in nursing personnel and to assist personnel to carry them out.

To accomplish this, the MacDonald House staff development program has four major areas of effort. These are (1) basic orientation of new employees, (2) follow-up of orientation and workshop participation, (3) providing opportunities for individuals or groups to improve their nursing skills or their understanding and approach to a nursing care situation, and (4) assistance with implementation of new programs or of new approaches to current programs.

Goals

1. Full implementation of the MacDonald House orientation program

*Courtesy University Hospitals of Cleveland, Cleveland, Ohio.

2. Completion of the revised MacDonald House orientation manual
3. Preparation and use of written orientation guides on all divisions similar to the one now in use on the fourth floor
4. Continued and more thorough follow-up of individuals
5. Creation of a master plan of experiences, etc. that should be provided for all individuals currently employed in MacDonald House and implementation of such a plan
6. Continued new learning opportunities for nursing staff such as the following:
   a. Neonatal hyperbilirubinemia and nursing care in phototherapy
   b. The adolescent mother
   c. The grieving process
   d. Assessment of pain and appropriate nursing intervention
   e. Mother-infant bonding
   f. Hysterectomy nursing care
   g. Types of anesthesia and nursing care considerations
7. Continued responsiveness to the needs of divisions and individuals
8. Formation of an ongoing MacDonald House staff development committee comprised of senior clinical nurses, nurse clinicians, supervisors, the assistant director, and the assistant instructor for staff development, the purpose of which would be to regularly evaluate and modify the staff development program in MacDonald House

Exhibit E

DEPARTMENT OF NURSING EDUCATION*

Philosophy

The faculty of the Department of Nursing Education at William Beaumont Hospital believes that quality individualized care of patients will be the primary goal toward which all hospital activities are directed. To be effective, the staff of the Department of Nursing Education must move in unison with the hospital's total plan of operation.

It is held by the nursing education faculty that within every employee there is an underlying and continuous need and right to learn that which is essential to satisfactory performance, according to his assigned position description. It is also believed that an ever-changing technology and the acquisition of new knowledge affecting the care of patients require an active continuing education program to maintain and upgrade the quality of nursing care. It is further believed that the increasing specialization and segregation of nursing and medical care services dictate that the learning needs of the nursing staff on each unit are best identified and provided for by the key result nursing staff members assigned to each unit in on-site unit teaching programs. The faculty of the Nursing Education Department expects to assume the responsibility of sharing in individual ward teaching classes by making available its consultation service and teaching facilities, equipment, and materials and by direct participation.

The faculty also holds the conviction that while provision for education of the nursing

*Courtesy William Beaumont Hospital, Royal Oak, Mich.

staff is its major responsibility, the special contributions of members of other health disciplines are necessary for an integrated curriculum. Therefore, because we support these beliefs, the Department of Nursing Education faculty makes a commitment to provide leadership for staff development, both individually and collectively, through the provision and support of educational activities. It is expected that these activities, based on the specific learning needs of the nursing personnel, will subsequently result in improved quality of patient care and increased job satisfaction and is one means through which progress is made.

Purpose

The purpose of the nursing education program is to provide opportunities for employed nursing personnel to acquire the knowledge, understanding, and skills necessary to safely and effectively perform the functions specified in their assigned position descriptions. It is also the purpose of the Department of Nursing Education to provide effective liaison between the Clinical Nursing Service Department and affiliating nursing student groups who utilize the hospital's clinical nursing facilities and other hospital departments for purposes of education.

Toward these purposes the following objectives are identified.

Objectives

1. To identify learning needs and to plan and implement teaching activities designed to assist those who come without preservice

preparation to function safely and effectively in their specific areas of assignment

2. To plan and implement centralized classes that will introduce those with preservice nursing education to those general nursing policies and procedures that are necessary for an orientation to their assigned positions

3. To assist in the provision of opportunities for continued learning that will assist nursing employees to keep abreast of an ever-changing body of knowledge affecting the care of patients to whom they are assigned

4. To plan and implement classes for key result nursing personnel designed to maintain and upgrade effective supervision and teaching skills required in the management of patient care and in the provision of unit teaching classes

5. To form positive working relationships with clinical nursing service personnel for the purpose of increasing effective communications and for the mutual benefit of the nursing staff and patients

6. To provide effective liaison between the nursing staff of this hospital and the nursing school faculty and students who utilize the clinical facilities in order that the affiliating students will be provided with meaningful learning experiences without hazards to the safety of patients

7. To advise the medical librarian of appropriate sources of nursing reference textbooks and periodicals suitable for permanent acquisition by the library

8. To acquire and/or develop current audiovisual materials and to make them known and available to the entire nursing staff and to the staff of other departments as requested

9. To assist the clinical nursing coordinator to identify the usual daily nursing care problems for the purpose of designing a meaningful orientation plan

10. To provide each clinical nursing coordinator with ongoing assistance, consultation, or direct participation in the planning and implementation of unit teaching

Exhibit F

MODEL FOR DECENTRALIZED STAFF DEVELOPMENT OFFERING*

Material presented in decentralized staff development sessions for nursing personnel in a specific hospital setting is based on the results of clinical research conducted by nurses and physicians and should reflect the current nursing and medical practice in the particular institution.

SESSIONS ON NEWBORN RESUSCITATION IN THE POSTPARTUM NURSERY
Preparation

How and why planned:

Requested by nursing personnel on postpartum divisions who felt they lacked the necessary skills to function efficiently when a newborn was in apparent respiratory difficulty, dates and times were discussed in advance with senior clinical nurses and supervisors involved.

Persons to attend:

All RN's and LPN's on postpartum and newborn units who have previously attended class on nursing assessment of the newborn and have had supervised practice in newborn assessment.

Purposes:

1. To familiarize nursing personnel with basic principles and procedures of newborn resuscitation, especially as they apply to the apparently healthy newborn in a postpartum nursery
2. To provide an opportunity for personnel to practice the procedures

Objectives:

Short term—by the end of the session participants will:

*Courtesy University Hospitals of Cleveland, Cleveland, Ohio; prepared by Susan Horsfall, R.N., B.S.N., Assistant Instructor, Maternity and Gynecology Nursing, University Hospitals, Cleveland, Ohio.

1. Describe verbally the criteria for evaluating the cardiopulmonary status of a newborn.
2. Discuss proper sequence of events during an emergency situation.
3. Demonstrate competency in the following procedures:
   a. Suction with bulb
   b. Suction with catheter
   c. Administration of oxygen
   d. Artificial ventilation—bag breathing
   e. External cardiac massage
4. State verbally the location of all emergency equipment and drugs that might be used for resuscitation of a newborn.

Long-term: Function effectively and efficiently when an infant needs emergency resuscitative care.

Methods:

1. Lecture/discussion of principles and procedures
   a. Ask group to list symptoms that indicate presence of excess secretion or airway obstruction.
   b. Ask group to indicate reasons why prolonged or overvigorous suctioning may be harmful.
   c. Have group list items to include when writing nurse's notes following suctioning.
   d. Have group list items to include when charting during a major resuscitative effort.

2. Demonstration of procedures
   a. Bulb suctioning with weighted doll
   b. Suctioning with catheter and Gomco aspirator
   c. Administration of oxygen using weighted doll and mask alone and bag and mask
   d. Artificial ventilation of model with gauges using mask and bag
   e. Cardiac compression using weighted doll
3. Return demonstration by all participants in the above procedures

Materials:
1. Bulb syringes, disposable and nondisposable
2. Suction catheters, plastic, sizes 8 and 10
3. Paper cup with water
4. Small bottle of sterile, distilled water
5. Gomco aspirator
6. Weighted doll, size of newborn
7. Model of newborn head with gauges and bellows attached
8. Oxygen tank with liter meter and bubble bottle
9. Newborn mask and bag
10. Newborn emergency trays

REFERENCES

Behrman, R. E., James, L. S., Klaus, M., Nelson, N., and Oliver, T.: Treatment of the asphyxiated newborn infant, J. Pediatr. **74:**981, 1969.

Gruber, H. S., and Klaus, M. H.: Intermittent mask and bag therapy, J. Pediatr. **76:**195, 1970.

Oropharyngeal aspiration of newborn, University Hospitals Nursing Council Policy No. 4 with Maternity and Gynecology Guidelines.

Roberts, J. E.: Suctioning the newborn, Am. J. Nurs. **73:**63, 1973.

Outline of content: lecture/discussion material*

I. Determining the need—assessing the patient
   A. Mucus within normal or expected limits
      1. Most normal full-term infants are capable of handling small amounts of mucus themselves.
         a. Natural reflexes to do this include swallowing, gagging, and coughing.

*Includes only a sample of the content.

   b. Infants should be propped on their sides to facilitate the natural process and to prevent choking; support should extend the full length of the back and include the head to prevent the baby's turning over.
   2. Only after the baby has been positioned on its side and respirations assessed should further measures be considered.
      a. If respiratory rate is within normal limits (40 to 60/min), without difficulty, slightly irregular but quiet, and the infant's color pink to red, the infant is successfully handling his own secretions.
      b. If respirations and infant's color deviate from normal or are indicative of difficulty, then further measures are necessary.
   3. Sneezing and coughing are the natural, normal methods by which an infant clears its nostrils of mucus, dust, etc. It does not mean the baby has a cold!
   B. Symptoms that indicate presence of excess secretions or airway obstruction and that indicate a need for suction (Ask group to list—add as necessary.)
      1. Obvious secretions in mouth and/or nose
      2. Noisy respirations—grunting, wheezing, stertorous
      3. Flaring of nares
      4. Air hunger with gasping respirations
      5. Irregular respirations
         a. Periods of apnea
         b. Rapid, shallow respirations
         c. Seesaw respirations
      6. Retractions
         a. Intercostal
         b. Substernal
         c. Clavicular
      7. Cyanosis of face and body
   C. Action taken depends on severity of symptoms
II. Basic resuscitative measures

Exhibit G

CENTRALIZED ORIENTATION PROGRAM FOR REGISTERED NURSES*

Policies

1. Centralized orientation classes will extend over a three-week period. Decentralized orientation will continue as long as necessary.
2. The first four weeks will be spent on the day tour of duty. Exceptions will be made by the assistant director.
3. Hours of duty should be scheduled to allow for attendance at classes during duty hours.
4. Attendance at all classes is required and planned in collaboration with the assistant director with the following exceptions:
   a. Reinstated registered nurses—attendance at classes will be decided on an individual basis.
   b. Part-time registered nurses—will be expected to attend as many of the classes as possible.

Purpose

Assist the registered nurse to become acquainted with the responsibilities of her role as determined by her position category and help her feel secure in the working environment of the University Medical Center.

Objectives†

Given the opportunity to attend orientation classes, observe demonstrations, and practice, the newly employed registered nurse at University Hospitals will be able by the end of the basic centralized orientation program to:

*Courtesy University Hospitals of Cleveland, Cleveland, Ohio; from Nursing Organization Manual, May, 1973.
†Only a portion of the total objectives are cited.

1. Recognize own position in the specific clinical area within the overall organizational structure of the Department of Nursing.
2. Recognize the position of the director, assistant director, nurse clinician, and senior clinical nurse in the organizational structure in own clinical area.
3. Recognize the joint relationship between the School of Nursing and the Department of Nursing at University Hospitals, the role of the nurse clinician, and the redefinition of role expectations of nursing personnel.
4. Recognize the availability and purpose of the following manuals: *Nursing Practice Guidelines, Nursing Organization Manual, Administrative Policies and Procedures,* and *Hospital Policies and Routines.*
5. Recognize the purpose and functions of the Nursing Council as outlined in Nursing Council Policy No. 1.
6. Recall the philosophy and objectives of the Department of Nursing as outlined in the *Nursing Organization Manual.*
7. Recall selected personnel policies as defined in "Rules and Procedures, Department of Nursing" and the *Administrative Policies and Procedures* manual.
8. Recall the philosophy, purpose, and objectives of staff development as outlined in the *Nursing Organization Manual.*
9. Identify the availability of library facilities.
10. Identify the role of the registered nurse in cardiopulmonary resuscitation.

a. Demonstrate appropriate cardiopulmonary resuscitation techniques on "Resusci-Anne."

b. Recognize the role of supporting personnel in cardiopulmonary resuscitation.

11. Identify the role and legal responsibilities of the registered nurse concerning the administration of medications as outlined in Nursing Council Policy No. 5 and related guidelines.

a. Recall the role of the registered nurse in the transcription of medication orders.

b. Recall the established procedure for the administration of medications.

c. Demonstrate the established procedures for recording medications.

d. Recall the role and legal responsibilities of the licensed practical nurse and nursing assistant in the administration of medications.

12. Recognize the use of selected work sheets used on the patient divisions to plan and record nursing care.

13. Identify the role and legal responsibilities of the registered nurse concerning intravenous therapy as outlined in Nursing Council Policy No. 5 and related guidelines.

a. Demonstrate the correct use of intravenous solutions and equipment, including hyperalimentation.

b. Recall the proper procedure for administration of medications via the intravenous route.

c. Recall the role and legal responsibilities of the licensed practical nurse and nursing assistant in intravenous therapy.

14. Recall the basic principles and demonstrate the proper technique involved in central venous pressure monitoring as outlined in Nursing Council Policy No. 6 and related guidelines.

15. Recall the role of the registered nurse concerning treatments and procedures related to the respiratory system as described in Nursing Council Policy No. 5 and related guidelines.

a. Demonstrate the proper use of suctioning equipment.

b. Recall the various types of intratracheal equipment and the nursing care involved with each.

c. Recognize and demonstrate the use of selected equipment used in inhalation therapy.

d. Recall and demonstrate the techniques used in teaching patients proper breathing exercises.

16. Discuss the role expectations for the registered nurse as outlined in the *Nursing Organizational Manual*.

a. Recall the major factors involved in changing titles and delineating role expectations for registered nurses with varying educational backgrounds.

b. Recognize how to identify own level of performance within the role description.

c. Recognize the role of the clinical nurse II as specified within the role description.

• • •

(Content and evaluation methods not included.)

RN CENTRALIZED ORIENTATION CLASS CALENDAR*

	MONDAY	TUESDAY	WEDNESDAY	THURSDAY	FRIDAY
Week #1	Room ____ 8:45-3:00 Orientation to University Hospitals Dept. of Nursing 3:00-4:00 Chest x-ray Lab work	Room ____ 8:30-1:30 University Hospitals orientation (meet in Personnel Dept. at 8:20) 1:30 Escort to assigned division	Room ____ Report to division at appropriate starting time 10:00-12:00 Class Emergencies 12:00-1:00 Lunch 1:00 Division practice	Room ____ A.M. Division practice 10:00-12:00 Class Medication policies 12:00-1:00 Lunch 1:00 Division practice	Room ____ A.M. Division practice Lunch—as assigned 1:00-3:45 Class IV therapy CVP Hyperalimentation
Week #2	Room ____ A.M. Division practice Lunch—as assigned 1:00-3:45 Class Suctioning Inhalation therapy	Room ____ A.M. Division practice Lunch—as assigned 1:30-3:45 Class RN role description Team nursing guidelines	Room ____ A.M. Division practice Lunch—as assigned 1:30-3:45 Class Role descriptions—other nursing staff Teaching programs Paramedical services	Room ____ A.M. Experience with Div. Coord. Lunch—as assigned 2:00-3:45 Class Division Coordinator program	Room ____ On division or Day off
Week #3	Room ____ On division or Day off	Room ____ A.M. Division practice Lunch—as assigned 2:00-3:45 Class Fire program, part 1 Hospital safety	Room ____ A.M. Division practice Lunch—as assigned 2:00-3:45 Class Fire program, part 2	Room ____ A.M. Division practice Lunch—as assigned 2:00-3:45 Class Legal responsibilities Community resources Evaluation of orientation	Room ____ On division or Day off

*Space for date provided in upper left-hand corner.

Exhibit H

CENTRALIZED ORIENTATION PROGRAM FOR LICENSED PRACTICAL NURSES*

Policies

1. Centralized orientation classes will extend over a three-week period. After this, planned decentralized orientation will continue as long as necessary on the division.
2. The first three weeks will be spent on the day tour of duty. Exceptions will be made by the assistant director.
3. Hours of duty should be scheduled to allow for attendance at classes during duty hours.
4. Attendance at all classes is required and planned in collaboration with the assistant director with the following exceptions.
   a. Reinstated licensed practical nurses—attendance at classes will be decided on an individual basis.
   b. Part-time licensed practical nurses—will be expected to attend as many of the classes as possible.
   c. Licensed practical nurses working in Rainbow Babies and Children operating room/recovery room and Hanna Pavilion 2 are not required to attend the math classes in week three.

Purpose

Assist the licensed practical nurse to become acquainted with her role and responsibilities in accordance with her position description and help her feel secure in the working environment of the University Medical Center.

*Courtesy University Hospitals of Cleveland, Cleveland, Ohio; from Nursing Organization Manual, May, 1973.

Objectives*

Given the opportunity to attend orientation classes, observe demonstrations, and practice, the newly employed licensed practical nurse at University Hospitals will be able by the end of the basic centralized orientation program to:

1. Recognize own position in the specific clinical area within the overall organizational structure of the Department of Nursing.
2. Recognize the position of the director, assistant director, nurse clinician, and senior clinical nurse in the organizational structure in own clinical area.
3. Recognize the joint relationship between the School of Nursing and the Department of Nursing at University Hospitals, the role of the nurse clinician, and the redefinition of role expectations of nursing personnel.
4. Recognize the availability and purpose of the following manuals: *Nursing Practice Guidelines, Nursing Organization Manual, Administrative ·Policies and Procedures*, and *Hospital Policies and Routines*.
5. Recognize the purpose and functions of the Nursing Council as outlined in Nursing Council Policy No. 1.
6. Recall the philosophy and objectives of the Department of Nursing as outlined in the *Nursing Organization Manual*.
7. Recall selected personnel policies as defined in "Rules and Procedures, Depart-

*Only a portion of the total objectives are cited.

ment of Nursing" and the *Administrative Policies and Procedures* manual.

8. Recall the philosophy, purpose, and objectives of staff development as outlined in the *Nursing Organization Manual.*

9. Identify the availability of library facilities.

10. Recognize the services available to patients by various paramedical departments.

11. Identify the role of the licensed practical nurse in cardiopulmonary resuscitation.
    a. Demonstrate appropriate cardiopulmonary resuscitation techniques on "Resusci-Anne."
    b. Recognize the role of the registered nurse and supporting personnel in cardiopulmonary resuscitation.

12. Identify the overall role expectations for licensed practical nurses as described in the *Nursing Organization Manual.*

13. Recognize the importance of a systematic approach to evaluation of nursing personnel.
    a. Recognize the existence of a performance evaluation for licensed practical nurses as specified in the *Nursing Organization Manual.*
    b. Recognize the relationship of the performance evaluation to the role description.
    c. Discuss the concept of self-evaluation as a part of the overall process.

14. Demonstrate awareness of role expectations of other classifications of nursing personnel.

15. Discuss the philosophy and concepts of "Guidelines for Team Nursing" as outlined in the *Nursing Organization Manual,* which includes sections on delegation and accountability, nursing care, teaching and learning, performance appraisal, and safety and environment.

16. Recall guidelines for recording clear, concise, and pertinent nurses' notes.

17. Recognize the use of selected work sheets used on the patient division to plan and record nursing care.

18. Identify the legal responsibilities of the licensed practical nurse and discuss the procedure for incident reporting.

19. Recognize the formal and informal educational opportunities available in the community and the University Medical Center for personal and vocational growth and development.

20. Recognize the purpose and availability of the local, state, and national organizations established for licensed practical nurses.

• • •

(Content and evaluation methods not included.)

LPN CENTRALIZED ORIENTATION CLASS CALENDAR*

	MONDAY	TUESDAY	WEDNESDAY	THURSDAY	FRIDAY
	Room ———	Room ———	Room ———	Room ———	Room ———
Week #1	8:45-3:00 Orientation to University Hospitals Dept. of Nursing 3:00-4:00 Chest x-ray Lab work	8:30-1:30 University Hospitals orientation (meet in Personnel Dept. at 8:20) 1:30 Escort to assigned division	Report to division at appropriate starting time 10:00-12:00 Class Emergencies 12:00-1:00 Lunch 1:00 Division practice	On division or Day off	A.M. Division practice 10:00-12:00 Class LPN role description Team nursing guidelines Nursing records Legal responsibilities 12:00-1:00 Lunch 1:00 Division practice
	Room ———	Room ———	Room ———	Room ———	Room ———
Week #2	A.M. Division practice Lunch—as assigned 1:00-3:45 Class Suctioning Inhalation therapy	A.M. Division practice 10:00-12:00 Class Personal care of patients Related procedures 12:00-1:00 Lunch 1:00 Division practice	A.M. Division practice 10:00-12:00 Class Sterile technique Urinary care Related procedures 1:00 Division practice	On division or Day off	A.M. Division practice 10:00-12:00 Class IV therapy CVP 12:00-1:00 Lunch 1:00 Division practice
	Room ———	Room ———	Room ———	Room ———	Room ———
Week #3	A.M. Division practice Lunch—as assigned 1:00-2:00 Class Mathematics 2:00 Division practice	A.M. Division practice Lunch—as assigned 1:00-2:00 Class Mathematics 2:00-3:45 Class Fire program, part 1 Hospital safety	A.M. Division practice Lunch—as assigned 1:00-2:00 Class Mathematics 2:00-3:45 Class Fire program, part 2 Evaluation of orientation	A.M. Division practice Lunch—as assigned 1:00-2:00 Class Mathematics 2:00 Division practice	On division or Day off

*Space for date provided in upper left-hand corner.

Exhibit I

CENTRALIZED ORIENTATION AND SKILL TRAINING SCHEDULE FOR NURSES' TECHNICAL ASSISTANT*

Week one

DAY	TIME	LOCATION AND TOPIC OF DISCUSSION
Sunday Date: _____	Day off	

Monday
Date: _____
	8:00 A.M.
	8:15-10:00
	
	10:00-12:00
	
	12:00-1:00
	1:00-4:30
		Meet instructors at Personnel Department
		Lockers
		Uniforms
		Harvey Conference Room A
		   Welcome
		   Objectives and philosophy
		   Personnel policies
		   Job description
		Lunch
		Harvey Conference Room A
		   Fire prevention
		   Introduction to patient units
		   Open bed demonstration—
		      return demonstration

Tuesday
Date: _____
	8:00 A.M.
	8:15-12:00
	
	12:00-1:00
	1:00-4:30
		Harvey Conference Room A
		Hanna Pavilion Ampitheater
		   University Hospitals orientation
		Lunch
		Harvey Conference Room A
		   Practice open bed making
		   Introduction to patient care
		   Bed bath demonstration—special
		      mouth care
		   Occupied bed demonstration—
		      return demonstration
		   Introduction to MTR (medical
		      treatment record)

Wednesday
Date: _____
	8:00-12:00
	
	12:00-12:45
		Division practice (under supervision
		    of instructor)
		   Beds
		Lunch

*Courtesy University Hospitals of Cleveland, Cleveland, Ohio; from Nursing Organization Manual, March, 1973.

Continued.

Week one—cont'd

DAY	TIME	LOCATION AND TOPIC OF DISCUSSION
	12:45-4:30	Harvey Conference Room A Study time Nutrition, diets, feeding patients, measuring and recording fluid, I&O Water pitchers

Thursday
Date: _____
	8:00-12:00	Division practice (under supervision
		    of instructor)
		Continuation of practice of duties
		    learned in classes to date

	12:00-12:45	Lunch

	12:45-4:30	Harvey Conference Room A
		Study time
		Physical therapist lecture—positioning,
		    transferring, ambulation
		Instructor—return demonstration
		    of ROM, bed attachments,
		    manipulation, traction
		Safety—patient and employee

Friday
Date: _____
	8:00-1:00	Division practice (under supervision
		    of instructor)
		Beds, personal care, feeding patients,
		    I&O, water pitchers

	1:00-1:45	Lunch
	1:45-4:30	Harvey Conference Room A Study time Special back care, decubitus prevention Ace bandages and elastic stockings Footboards and cradles, CD demonstration Urosheath and peri-care, MTR
Saturday Date: _____	Day off	

Week two

DAY	TIME	LOCATION AND TOPIC OF DISCUSSION
Sunday Date: _____	Day off	

Monday
Date: _____
	8:00-1:00	Division practice (under supervision
		    of instructor)
		Beds, personal care, Ace bandages,
		    decubitus care, feeding patients
		I&O, water pitchers

	1:00-1:45	Lunch
	1:45-4:30	Harvey Conference Room A Study time Specimen collecting

Week two—cont'd

DAY	TIME	LOCATION AND TOPIC OF DISCUSSION
Tuesday Date: _____	8:00-1:00	Division practice (under supervision of instructor) Beds, personal care, feeding patients Specimen collection I&O, water pitchers
	1:00-1:45	Lunch

	1:45-4:30	Harvey Conference Room A
		    Tour of labs
		    Review specimens

Wednesday Date: _____	8:00-1:00	Division practice (under supervision of instructor) Beds, personal care, feeding patients I&O, specimen collection
	1:00-1:45	Lunch

	1:45-4:30	Harvey Conference Room A
		    Study time
		    TPR theory and practice

Thursday
Date: _____
	8:00-1:00	Division practice (under supervision
		    of instructor)
		Practice of all duties listed above
		    with emphasis on TPR

	1:00-1:45	Lunch

	1:45-4:30	Harvey Conference Room A
		    Study time
		    Blood pressure theory and practice

Friday
Date: _____
	8:00-11:00	Harvey Conference Room A
		    Charting
		    Housekeeping

	11:00-11:45	Lunch

	11:45-2:00	Harvey Conference Room A
		    Study time
		    Conferences

	2:00-4:30	Division practice (under supervision
		    of instructor)
		Sterilizing, discharge units, utility
		    room, division housekeeping

Saturday Date: _____	Day off	

Week three

DAY	TIME	LOCATION AND TOPIC OF DISCUSSION
Sunday Date: _____	Day off	
Monday Date: _____	8:00-12:00	Division practice (under supervision of instructor)
	12:00-12:45	Lunch

Continued.

Week three—cont'd

DAY	TIME	LOCATION AND TOPIC OF DISCUSSION

	12:45-4:30	Harvey Conference Room A
		Admission of patients
		    Attitudes and behaviors
		    Admission procedures

Tuesday
Date: _____
	1:00-5:15	Harvey Conference Room A
		Preoperative care
		    Enema theory
		    Demonstration and practice
		    Skin prep, bed, personal care
		    Evening care

	5:15-6:00	Dinner

	6:00-9:30	Division practice (under supervision
		    of instructor)
		    Preoperative care, evening care

Wednesday
Date: _____
	1:00-5:15	Harvey Conference Room A
		Postoperative care
		    Binders
		    Sitz bath
		    IV's
		    Oxygen therapy
		    Hot-water bottle
		    Ice cap

	5:15-6:00	Dinner

	6:00-9:30	Division practice (under supervision
		    of instructor)
		    Evening care, postoperative care

Thursday Date: _____	Day off	

Friday
Date: _____
	8:00-12:00	Division practice (under supervision
		    of instructor)
		    Practice of duties taught to date

	12:00-12:45	Lunch

	12:45-3:00	Harvey Conference Room A
		    Diagnostic tests, messenger duties
		    Tour of messenger areas
		    Study time

	3:00-4:30	Conferences
Saturday Date: _____	7:00-3:45	Division practice (under supervision of instructor)

Week four (review and classroom make-up as necessary)

DAY	TIME	LOCATION AND TOPIC OF DISCUSSION
Sunday Date: _____	7:00-3:45	Division practice (under supervision of instructor)
Monday Date: _____	7:00-3:45	Training division practice

Week four—cont'd

DAY	TIME	LOCATION AND TOPIC OF DISCUSSION
Tuesday Date: _____	7:00-3:45	Training division practice
Wednesday Date: _____	Day off	
Thursday Date: _____	7:00-1:00 1:00-1:45 1:45-3:45	Training division practice Lunch Harvey Conference Room A 　Team nursing concept
Friday Date: _____	7:00-12:00 12:00-12:45 12:45-3:45	Training division practice Lunch Harvey Conference Room A 　Emergencies 　Equipment 　Telepage (triple) 　"Mr. Strong" 　"Dr. Fuse" 　Tour of assigned division
Saturday Date: _____	Day off	

Week five (review and classroom make-up as necessary)

DAY	TIME	LOCATION AND TOPIC OF DISCUSSION
Sunday Date: _____	Day off	
Monday Date: _____	7:00-3:45	Own division practice
Tuesday Date: _____	7:00-3:45	Own division practice
Wednesday Date: _____	7:00-12:00 12:00-12:45 12:45-3:45	Own division practice Lunch Harvey Conference Room A 　Study time 　Isolation 　　Theory 　　Procedure 　　Demonstration and practice
Thursday Date: _____	7:00-12:00 12:00-12:45 12:45-3:45	Own division practice Lunch Harvey Conference Room A 　After-death care 　　Theory and demonstration 　Tour of morgue

Continued.

Week five—cont'd

DAY	TIME	LOCATION AND TOPIC OF DISCUSSION
Friday Date: _____	7:00-12:00 12:00-12:45 12:45-3:45	Own division practice Lunch Harvey Conference Room A Final exam
Saturday Date: _____	Day off	

Week six

DAY	TIME	LOCATION AND TOPIC OF DISCUSSION
Sunday Date: _____	Day off	
Monday Date: _____	7:00-12:00 12:00-12:45 12:45-3:45	Own division practice Lunch Harvey Conference Room A Review Checklists Shift duties Evaluations Staff development activities
Tuesday Date: _____	*Scheduled by division	Follow-up by instructors as needed

*Trainee should be scheduled to work on Saturday of sixth week on roll.

Exhibit J

ORIENTATION AND SKILL TRAINING CLASS FOR NURSES' TECHNICAL ASSISTANT*

Subject: Physical therapy and body mechanics

Outline: I. Demonstration by physical therapist
II. Discussion of transfer techniques
III. Bed positioning
IV. Ambulating
V. Range of motion

Audiovisual aids

Bulletin board

Filmstrips: "Positioning to Prevent Contractures" and "Transfer Activities and Ambulation"

Equipment

Restraints
Robe with belt, slippers
Ice bag with cover
Stretcher (from EW)
Wheelchair (in classroom)

Objectives

The NTA trainee will:

1. Be able to move patients safely from bed to chair, chair to bed, and stretcher to bed and to ambulate patients.
2. Be aware of and use good body mechanics.
3. Prevent the patients' development of contractures by good positioning and by using range of motion exercises.
4. Know how to apply restraints.

REFERENCES

Cherescavich, G.: A textbook for nursing assistants, ed. 3, St. Louis, 1973, The C. V. Mosby Co., chaps. 12 and 13.
Training the nursing aids, Chicago, 1969, Hospital Research & Educational Trust, chaps. 13 and 14.

*Courtesy University Hospitals of Cleveland, Cleveland, Ohio.

Leake, M.: A manual of simple nursing procedures, Philadelphia, 1971, W. B. Saunders Co., chap. 5.

Content

I. Demonstration by physical therapist
  A. Transferring patients
    1. Bed ←→ Chair
    2. Bed ←→ Stretcher
    3. Three-man lift
    4. Two-man lift
II. Discussion of transfer techniques
  A. Purpose
    1. Types of patients
      a. CVA
      b. Paraplegic
      c. Postoperative
      d. Injured foot
      e. Helpless
        (1) Parkinsonism
        (2) Arthritic
  B. Safety measures
  C. Stress good side out
  D. Body mechanics
    1. Lifting—feet apart, knees bent, back straight, weight close to body; lift by straightening legs; bend knees when putting weight down
  E. Practice
  F. Filmstrip: "Positioning to Prevent Contractures"
III. Bed positioning
  A. Purpose
  B. Precautions
  C. Demonstration of different positions
    1. Supine
    2. Prone

3. Side-lying
4. Fowler's
5. Trendelenberg
D. Turning and moving up in bed
E. Use of side rails and cord
F. Dangling
G. Practice
IV. Ambulating
  A. Purpose
  B. Safety measures
    1. Proper slippers
      a. Shoelaces tied

      2. Faint, wobbly
      3. Stumbling over furniture
      4. Robe with belt
  C. Demonstration
  D. Practice
V. Range of motion
  A. Purpose
  B. Precautions
  C. Demonstration
    1. Upper extremity
    2. Lower extremity
  D. Practice

Exhibit K

LEADERSHIP DEVELOPMENT WORKSHOP*†

SN II BASIC
SESSION I—A.M.

Introduction: Discussion of workshop purposes, references, and assignments

Assignment: Review attached role description for SN II's.

Bring this role description to each workshop session.

Following introduction, morning will be used for library work and individual assignments.

SESSION I—P.M.

Topic

"The Leader and the Work Group."

Objectives

1. Identify leader behaviors and their application to the clinical area by analyzing a videotape using Lippett and White's classification of leader style.
2. Apply leader behaviors to the team leader's functions of delegating and holding nursing staff accountable.
3. Relate principles of leadership to the work group in the clinical area.

Assignment

None.

REFERENCES

°Babnew, D.: The whys' of wise delegation, Hospitals **39**:62, July, 1965.

Cartwright, D., and Zander, A.: Group dynamics, New York, 1968, Harper & Row, Publishers, pp. 91-105, 192-198, °301-315, 318-355, 389-398.

°Frazier, L. M.: Accountability: third essential in process of delegation, Hosp. Top. **44**:81, June, 1966.

Holloman, C. R.: Leadership and headship: there is a difference, Notes and Quotes, January, 1971.

Krech, D., Crutchfield, R. S., and Ballachey, E. I.: Individual in society, New York, 1962, McGraw-Hill Book Co., pp. 432-447.

Merton, R. K.: The social nature of leadership, Am. J. Nurs. **69**:2614, 1969.

°White, H. C.: Some perceived behavior and attitudes of hospital employees under effective and ineffective supervisors, J. Nurs. Admin. **1**(1):49, 1971.

°White, H. C.: Perceptions of leadership styles by nurses in supervisory positions, J. Nurs. Admin. **1**(2):44, 1971.

SN II BASIC
SESSION II—A.M.

Topic

"Observing and Recording Clinical Performance."

Objectives

1. Discuss principles basic to the process of evaluation of clinical performance.
2. Discuss the process of objective observation and recording of clinical performance.
3. View film "Eye of Beholder" and discuss how content relates to No. 2.
4. Criticize examples of anecdotal records for

°Courtesy University Hospitals of Cleveland, Cleveland, Ohio.

†Includes only a sample of total workshop syllabus.

°Read first.

objectivity and identify their significance in evaluating progress.

5. Discuss the role of the SN II for observing and recording performance.

6. Observe and record one actual instance of clinical performance during the week following the class and bring to the next class session.

Assignment

Be prepared to discuss system of performance appraisal on own division and expectations for self, particularly regarding anecdotal records.

REFERENCES

Barrett, J.: The head nurse, her changing role, ed. 2, New York, 1968, Appleton-Century-Crofts, chap. 18.

Mager, R.: Developing attitude toward learning, Belmont, Calif., 1968, Fearon Publishers, pp. 13-30.

Review "Role Expectations and Performance Evaluation" forms for NTA's, LPN's, and SN II's. (Refer to *Nursing Organization Manual,* section II: C9, C7, and C6, and section III: B5, B3, and B2, which is found at the nurses' station on each division)

Exhibit L

1972-1973 CENTRALIZED STAFF DEVELOPMENT SCHEDULE*

PROGRAM	Day	Time	AUG	SEPT	OCT	NOV	DEC	JAN	FEB	MAR	APR	MAY	JUNE	JULY
Orientation														
RN (CN I, SN II)	M		14, 28	11, 25	9, 23	6, 20	4, 18	2, 15, 29	12, 26	12, 26	9, 23	7, 21	4, 18	2, 16, 30
RN (SN I)	M		14	11, 25		6	18	15, 29			9, 23	7, 21		2, 16
LPN	M		14, 28	11, 25	9, 23	6, 20	4, 18	2, 15, 29	12, 26	12, 26	9, 23	7, 21	4, 18	2, 16, 30
NTA	M		7		30			8			2			
Continuing education RN's														
SN I (spec. pro. pt. 1)	Tu	1-4 8:30-4 1-4			3, 10, 17			9, 16, 23			10, 17, 24.			10, 17, 24
SN I (spec. pro. pt. 2)	Tu	8:30-4		5, 12, 19			5, 12, 19			6, 13, 20			5, 12, 19	
Sn II (basic)	W	8:30-4			18, 25	1, 29	6, 13	31	7, 14	14, 21, 28	25	2, 9		
SN II (promotional)	Th	8:30-4				2, 9, 16				1, 8, 15				
CN I (basic)	W	8:30-4			4, 11			10, 17, 24	21, 28	7	4, 11, 18	16, 23, 30		
CN I (promotional)	Tu	8:30-4			24, 31	7, 14					24	1, 8, 15		
SCN (basic)	F	8:30-4				3, 10, 17	15							
SCN (ongoing)	Th	8:30-4		14, 21		30	7		15, 22			3, 10		

*Courtesy University Hospitals of Cleveland, Cleveland, Ohio.

Continued.

1972-1973 CENTRALIZED STAFF DEVELOPMENT SCHEDULE—cont'd

PROGRAM	Day	Time	AUG	SEPT	OCT	NOV	DEC	JAN	FEB	MAR	APR	MAY	JUNE	JULY
LPN's LPN I (promotional)	Th	†			5, 12, 19, 26			Night tour 18, 25	1, 8	Evening tour 22, 29	5, 12			
LPN medication course					3 ——→ 17			16 ——————→ 7			3 ——→ 18			
NTA's NTA I (basic)	Tu	†		5, 12, 19, 26							On each tour of duty 24	1, 8		
NTA I (promotional)	Tu	†							Evening tour 13, 20, 27	6				
Div. coordinator program Supervisors (ongoing)	F	8:30-4				3, 10				2, 9				
Coordinators (basic)	F	8:30-12:30			6, 13, 20, 27					16, 23, 30	6			
Coordinators (ongoing)	Th F	8:30-4		28, 29							26, 27			
Drug fair				To be announced										
Equip. and supply Fair				To be announced										
Comm. Resources Fair				To be announced										

†Evening tour: 3:00-7:30 P.M. Night tour: 11:30-3:30 A.M.

Exhibit M

CALENDAR OF DECENTRALIZED STAFF DEVELOPMENT ACTIVITIES IN MATERNITY AND GYNECOLOGY NURSING SERVICE*

MARCH 1973

				1	2	3
4	5	6 "Continuity Prenatal Care Conference": Selected RN's from in- and outpatient services, 12:30 P.M. "Newborn Nursing Assessment": All personnel M6, 2:00 P.M.	7 "Breathing and Relaxation Techniques used in Labor": RN's and LPN's M4, 12:30-1:30 P.M.	8 "Team Leading": RN's M4-5, 8 A.M. "Newborn Nursing Assessment": RN's and LPN's 3:30-4:30 P.M.	9	10
11	12 "Recording Patient Data": RN's and LPN's, 1:00 P.M. "Pre-Op Teaching": RN's and LPN's, 10:15-11:15 A.M.	13	14 "Team Leading": RN's M4-5, 8:00 and 10:00 A.M.	15 "Care of Pregnant Diabetic During Labor": RN's and LPN's M6, 5:30-6:30 P.M.	16 "Pre-Op Teaching": RN's and LPN's 10:15-11:15 A.M.	17

*Courtesy University Hospitals of Cleveland, Cleveland, Ohio.

Continued.

MARCH 1973

18	19	20	21	22	23	24
		"Continuity Pre-natal Care Conference": Selected RN's from in- and outpatient services, 12:30-1:30 P.M. "Recording on Nurses' Notes": RN's and LPN's M4-5, 4:00 P.M.	"Recording on Nurse's Notes": RN's and LPN's, 10:15 A.M. "Role of Nursery Personnel in Newborn Resuscitation": RN's and LPN's, 3:30-4:30 P.M.		"Recording on Nurse's Notes": NTA's, 10:15 A.M. "Nursing Care Plans": RN's and LPN's M2, M4, M5, 1:00 A.M.	

25	26	27	28	29	30	31
	"Charting on Labor Records": RN's and LPN's, 7:30 A.M.	"Recording on Nurse's Notes": RN's and LPN's, 1:00 A.M; NTA's, 3:00 A.M.		"Pre-Op Teaching": RN's and LPN's, 4:15 P.M. "Recording on Nurse's Notes": RN's and LPN's, 1:00 A.M.; NTA's, 3:00 A.M.	"Charting on Labor Records": RN's and LPN's, 8:00 P.M.	

Exhibit N

LEADERSHIP DEVELOPMENT WORKSHOP*†

CN I PROMOTIONAL
SESSION II—A.M.

Topic

"Role of CN II in Performance Appraisal."

Objectives

1. Recognize the role of the CN II in evaluating the performance of others on the nursing team.
2. Review the principles and process of performance appraisal as needed.
3. Recognize existence, purpose, and content of a terminal summary.
4. Analyze the structure of evaluation forms for RN's, LPN's and NTA's, and compare and contrast major features such as terminology, degree of structure, use of rating scale, etc. (Small-group work.)
5. Describe specific examples of behavior that could be included in select categories outlined in the evaluation form. (Small-group work.)
6. Outline a long-range plan for working with a nursing staff member on own clinical division using the data mentioned in assignment. (Individual work.)

Assignment

Discuss with SCN the "system" for performance appraisal on own unit and your responsibility within the system. Bring to class all

data available (including previous evaluations and current anecdotal records) on one person with whom intensively working and for whom responsible.

REFERENCES

Albrecht, S.: Reappraisal of conventional performance appraisal systems, J. Nurs. Admin. 2(2):29, 1972.
Kimball, S., Pardee, G., and Larson, E.: Evaluation of staff performance, Am. J. Nurs. 71:1744, 1971.
McGregor, D.: An uneasy look at performance appraisal, Harvard Bus. Rev. 35(3):89, 1957.
Meyer, H. H., Kay, E., and French, J. R. P., Jr.: Split roles in performance appraisal, Harvard Bus. Rev. 43(1):45, 1965.
Palmer, M. E.: Self-evaluation of clinical performance, Nurs. Outlook 15:63, Nov., 1967.

CN I PROMOTIONAL
SESSION II—P.M.

Topic

"Guiding and Counseling Personnel."

Objectives

1. Discuss principles related to formal and informal counseling.
2. Review factors to consider when preparing for the counseling session.
3. Identify reasons for utilizing either a formal or an informal approach to counseling staff.
4. Demonstrate the use of these counseling principles in role-play situations.
5. Identify and discuss the dynamics of behaviors observed in role-play situations.

Assignment

Using the data gathered for the morning assignment, identify behaviors of the staff

---

*Courtesy University Hospitals of Cleveland, Cleveland, Ohio.

†Includes only a sample of total workshop syllabus.

members that would need to be discussed in a counseling situation. Decide on an approach you would use in counseling the individual—formal or on-the-spot counseling. Anticipate possible reactions he or she may have to the counseling session and plan your strategy for dealing with these reactions.

REFERENCES

Carlson, C. E.: Behavioral concepts and nursing intervention, Philadelphia, 1970, J. B. Lippincott Co., pp. 67-93.

Costly, D. L.: Basis for effective communication, Supervisor Nurse 4(1):16, 19, 1973.

Hobart, C. L.: The interview as a management skill, Supervisor Nurse 2(10):56, 1971.

Kolba, Sr. M. T.: The human equation in supervision, Supervisor Nurse 2(1):64, 67, 71, 1971.

Lysaught, J. P.: No carrots, no sticks: motivation in nursing, J. Nurs. Admin. 2(5):43, 1972.

O'Brien, M. J.: Evaluation: a positive, constructive approach to the development of potential, Supervisor Nurse 2(4):24, 1971.

Peplau, H.: Responsibility, authority, evaluation and accountability of nursing in patient care, Mich. Nurs. 44:5-7, 20-21, 23, July, 1971.

Exhibit O

CONTINUING EDUCATION* †

NTA I PROMOTIONAL

SESSION **II**

Topics

"Reporting and Recording Information" and "Interpersonal Relationship with Patient and Co-workers."

Objectives

1. Discuss means to improve NTA's skill in observing, reporting, and recording information pertaining to patients.
2. Identify knowledge of official hospital abbreviations and demonstrate ability to record pertinent information.

°Courtesy University Hospitals of Cleveland, Cleveland, Ohio.
†Includes only a sample of total workshop syllabus.

3. Identify attitudes that interfere with establishing positive interpersonal relationships with patients and co-workers.
4. Explore the NTA's role in relation to the division coordinators, secretaries, and the METS personnel.
5. View and discuss the film "Eye of the Beholder" and determine how participants can use this information in their daily encounters with patients, visitors, and staff.

Assignment

1. Complete patient care study.
2. Describe in writing a situation that occurred on your division that you would like to discuss with the person who is having follow-up conferences with you.

Exhibit P

GENERAL GUIDE TO EVALUATION OF STAFF DEVELOPMENT PROGRAMS

EVALUATION OF: Learners
Learning offering
Total staff development
effort

EVALUATION BASIS: Performance behaviors

Effects on learners during offering

1. Change in knowledge

2. Change in skill

3. Change in attitude

Effects on learners after offering

1. Change in behavior in terms of objectives

2. Change in competency and satisfaction

3. Change in needs (initial learning need was met by offering)

How to determine change

METHOD	POSITIVE INDICATORS
1. Pretests and Post-tests	1. Post-tests have higher scores.
2. Program evaluation	2. Positive feelings are expressed in writing.

3. Attendance record (not as significant with mandatory programs)

4. Participation

5. Interviews with significant others

6. Direct observation

7. Postprogram meetings

3. Learners have attended all or majority of classes.

4. Learners have participated in discussions.

5. Clinical superiors indicate change of behavior in accordance with expected outcomes.

6. Learners demonstrate use of new knowledge, skill, and attitude in simulated or clinical situation.

7. Learners relate how they used new knowledge, skill, and attitude in clinical situations.

Index